A POSTMORTEM OF GRIEF

ROBIN MCMURRY PHD, RNC

emerge
publishing

TULSA OKLAHOMA

25 24 23 22 21 20   9 8 7 6 5 4 3 2 1

A POSTMORTEM OF GRIEF:
Understanding the Emotional and Neurobiological Nature of Loss
Copyright ©2020 Robin McMurry, PhD, RNC

Published by:
Emerge Publishing, LLC
9521 Riverside Parkway, Suite 243 Tulsa, OK 74137
Phone: 888.407.4447
www.EmergePublishing.com

Cover Design by: Jarred Smith

Library of Congress Catalog-in-Publication Data:
ISBN: 978-1-949758-53-5 Paperback
ISBN: 978-1-949758-54-2 E-book
ISBN: 978-1-949758-55-9 Audiobook

BISAC:
FAM014000 FAMILY & RELATIONSHIPS / Death, Grief, Bereavement
PSY052000 PSYCHOLOGY / Grief & Loss
MED058200 MEDICAL / Nursing / Research & Theory

Printed in the United States

To my dad, Jim Archer, who loved us fiercely and left us too soon.

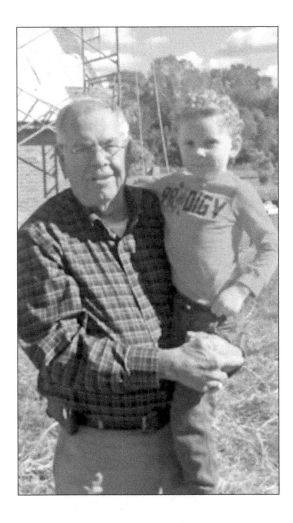

A POSTMORTEM OF GRIEF

There's a place in Peru where the sky meets the ground, and the atmosphere is so thin you can almost walk right out of oxygen.

That's what grief feels like.

TABLE OF CONTENTS

FALLING DOWN THE RABBIT HOLE

My dad is dead. For a long time after he died that's all I could write because the heaviness of that one sentence seemed as though the weight of the words alone would cause them to fall right through the paper. It was too painful to replay the images that I tried my best to repress. Somehow seeing these words in print made it final, as if his daily absence wasn't enough. I kept putting it off, shoving it to the back, hoping the urge to tell this story would pass and I would heal without ever having to relive even one minute of it. But telling the story helps to dissipate the pain. Reliving it often and in detail is primal to the grieving process. Grief must be witnessed to be healed.[1] So here I am, reluctantly sludging through this process, hoping healing will eventually come.

Throughout this ordeal, I keep thinking about *Alice in Wonderland*. I picture Alice falling headfirst down the rabbit hole, tumbling end over end through a long, black tunnel, the light from above fading as it gives way to a seemingly bottomless pit. It's dark and she continues to fall, bumping into things as she plunges deeper and deeper into the earth. Grief is a lot like that. So, I spend my days avoiding the rabbit hole. Staying as far away from the edge as I can. But that's hard to do, isn't it? And for those of us who crave control, it's a special kind of hell. Anything can send me tumbling down. In the movie, Alice wonders if she could fall straight through to the center of the earth. I wonder that, too. Maybe it's the falling down that I'm avoiding, or maybe it's never finding the bottom that I fear, and the writing of these words is only symbolic, and by proxy, a way to avoid the dark. Maybe I'm afraid that I will get so lost in grief that I won't be able to find my way back. Unlike Alice, I'm afraid of any bottle that says, "drink me," and yet, if I thought it would ease this pain, maybe I would.

His death was sudden. It happened on an ordinary day. There was no immediate warning that our lives were on a crash course with grief. In the aftermath, I kept thinking about being on a plane right before it crashes, when the pilot says, "Brace for impact." There was no announcement, no time to brace— just a sudden explosion and then nothing seemed familiar.

Nothing extraordinary about that day stood out, no warning that this would be the last conversation, the last picture, the last everything. It all came to a full stop. In her book *The Year of Magical Thinking*, Joan Didion writes of her husband's sudden death. "It was in fact the ordinary nature of everything preceding the event that prevented me from truly believing it had happened, absorbing it, incorporating it, getting past it."[2] I struggled with that, too. In the early days following his death, I would catch myself shaking my head as if to clear the confusion. It reminded me of the way television sets used to be. They would get poor reception, then wavy lines would appear on the screen. We would readjust the rabbit ears and bang on the side until, eventually, the picture became clear again. To clear my head, I would relive the sequence of events to make sure I understood what had taken place. Surely, there was something I was missing, something I just didn't understand. I had not the slightest idea how to cope with this new reality and my lack of experience with grief put me at a disadvantage.

While intellectually understanding death is easy, it takes much more time for it to finally penetrate the psyche. I once heard someone describe the immediate aftermath of the death of a friend. He said in the beginning, the loss is fluid. You may not have seen the person who died every day when they were alive, so you can pretend they are just gone, but at some point, you pass the timeframe when you would have ordinarily interacted with them, and that's when it begins to finally sink in. It takes a while for the loss to move from a liquid to a solid state. But eventually it does, and painfully so. It becomes more real. It's a process that must be worked through slowly, much like the freezing of water.

It's strange how one pivotal event can divide a life into two distinct segments so that everything is categorized into the before or after. An imaginary line separating one point in time from another. An abstract division. All preceding events are viewed through a new lens, one that is foggy at times and yet oddly clear. You suddenly know what matters, and you certainly know what doesn't.

There are eight nurses in my family. The subject of death, grief, and trauma are common to our profession. But this death was different. This death was personal. Grief is strange and unpredictable, and navigating it has been a minefield of pain, fear, gratitude, regret, and confusion. If death is black and white, then grief is gray. Some days are darker shades of gray and some days lighter, but the shades are always gray. If there's one thing I've learned about grief, it is the fact that it can only truly be understood from the inside out and, sometimes, not even then. This postmortem is an effort to understand my grief and maybe help my patients and their families understand theirs. Ultimately, my goal is to engage the medical community in a dialogue about preventive care of families in trauma, so we know how to effectively begin the healing process at the point of crisis, something not afforded us by some healthcare workers we encountered when my dad was dying.

What I have come to understand is this—everyone reacts differently when grief is their environment. It is rarely an easy transition, and while I am not given much to false starts, finding my path has been one of the most difficult things I have ever had to do. After living with this loss for a while now, bereavement remains somewhat of an enigma. It is important to me to capture the essence of this peculiar pain. The dissection of my grief is necessary for me to understand it. My dad would want me to look at the facts scientifically, to draw a conclusion, and to move on with my life. So, my response to grief led me to rely on my medical training as a nurse and researcher and dig deep into the data for answers, if they are to be found. This postmortem is an effort in that direction. Grief is at times overwhelming, but so is gratitude, and I am forever grateful to be his daughter.

CHAPTER ONE

AN ORDINARY DAY

When I arrive, I see him lying lifeless on the ground, one shoe is missing, his shirt is cut open, and his pants are ripped. There are two medical personnel at his head and one near his feet. I recognize the paramedic at his feet, and we lock eyes. His name is Jason. We grew up with him—went to the same church, our parents were friends, and his fire station is just down the street from my parents' house. I feel better that he is here. He knows my dad. I'm not sure why this brings me comfort, but it does. He is administering drugs to stabilize Dad's heart. They have performed a procedure called an intraosseous cannulation. They drill straight into the bone to administer medication. It's often used in emergency situations when quick access is necessary. As a clinician, I know what is happening; I understand the sequence of events involved in a resuscitation. This is familiar, and yet oddly foreign.

Everything I think I know about resuscitation swims around in my head, and I try to keep the sequence of events straight while I anticipate the next move. The clock is ticking and although the sound is not audible, I hear it in my head, and I know that precious seconds are slipping away—and so is he. It's difficult to think clinically in such a personal situation. That's why, as professionals, it's not best practice to treat those we love. When desperation enters the picture, it's hard to move emotion out of the way and think clearly when so much is personally on the line. It reminds me of what pilots must experience in an emergency, when the lives they are trying to save include their own. In my head, I move back and forth between differential diagnoses and emotional meltdown.

The intubation is rough and not successful on the first two attempts. My family is large, including eight nurses. By now, five of them are standing close by, wanting to help. But no one moves. We form a semicircle around the emergency workers and my dad's body. We are silent. The night is unseasonably warm for November and very calm despite the controlled chaos on the ground. The nurse in me wants to bark orders, but the daughter in me shrinks back in horror.

Much research has been done about family members being present during resuscitation. Allowing the family to be present means they are in a place where visual or physical contact with the patient is encouraged.[3] These studies have suggested it is beneficial to let families see, let them stay, let them witness that every effort is being made to save their loved one. But I can tell you—at least for me—watching this unfold is not helpful or in any way therapeutic. It is traumatizing, and the memory of it will linger. I will not be able to stop seeing his lifeless body on the ground. For some time, I will be unable to shake the feeling of desperation, panic, and the sheer horror of those fifteen minutes, and I will relive them—over and over.

For the first time in my life, I would come to understand on an intimate level what post-traumatic stress disorder (PTSD) really is. PTSD refers to the negative effects of exposure to stressful life events and the subsequent impact on the mental health of the individual.[4] Patients who experience PTSD may have recurrent memories of the traumatic event or may even relive it in the form of flashbacks, where they experience the trauma again and again. They may have nightmares and difficulty functioning during the day. For some patients, this process can be debilitating, and professional help may be needed to help them process the trauma. This "fallout" from traumatic events can make recovery difficult and prolonged.

It is dark, and the light from the garage shines into the night. My mother is standing nearby, and she shivers even though it is not cold. Her arms are wrapped tightly around her body as if she is physically holding herself together. She's wearing someone's coat around her shoulders. It's too big, which makes her look even more vulnerable. She is small, maybe five feet two, much shorter than my dad's six feet one. She tells us he was backing the truck into the garage when he slumped over the wheel. No words, no warning, he just ceased to be conscious. She got out of the truck and went around to his side. The truck, still running, rolled into the fence, breaking one of the wooden slats.

Somehow, she managed to pull him from the truck, call 911, and begin cardiopulmonary resuscitation (CPR) even though she has never been formally trained in the procedure. Through sheer force, she willed blood to flow again to his oxygen-deprived organs. I am still unclear how she managed to accomplish this, but somehow, she did. Later, she will also experience PTSD as she comes to grips with the weight of his death and her role in the resuscitation. Eventually, she will describe perfectly what PTSD is, even though I don't think she has ever labeled her experience with this acronym, and I don't think she understands its implication in delayed healing from trauma.

At the scene, my nephew has his arm around her, and he is explaining everything the paramedics are doing. His background is emergency medicine, and he understands the odds of success— or maybe more realistically, the odds of failure in these situations. Research tells us that only six percent of patients who experience out-of-hospital cardiac arrest (OHCA) will survive.[5] Statistics begin to flood my mind from past research I have read. Six percent. I repeat that to myself as numbers bounce around in my head. Six percent.

It's strange the things you think about during a crisis when time seems momentarily suspended. I remember a cooking show I once saw. The host (I forget now who she was) said "It matters what you bring to the party. If you want to have a good party, you need good ingredients." I have repeated this to my nursing students many times in relation to patients in the intensive care unit (ICU). It matters what they bring to the party. If the patient doesn't bring the good things (a disease-free heart, good kidneys, healthy lifestyle), they are less likely to survive. I look over at my dad's body and wonder how much good he is bringing. He's lived a clean lifestyle, mostly influenced by his strict religious beliefs. No drinking, no smoking, a healthy weight, but his genetics aren't good, and it's hard to outrun your genetics. He has already had two bypass surgeries, a few stints, and a couple of balloons. Even so, until a few minutes ago, he was active, brilliant, and alive, very much alive. Six percent: those words echo in my head like they have been yelled into the Grand Canyon.

I begin to remember every interaction I have ever had with desperate families of patients I have cared for and feel the weight of every death I have witnessed. These are the kinds of things we, as healthcare providers, try to push aside in our profession. We have to, if we are to be effective, able to go to the next bedside, and make sound clinical decisions. But on this night, the heaviness of all those traumas comes roaring back, and I feel I might suffocate under their weight. I feel like the oxygen is being sucked out of the universe.

I stare at my bare feet and gently move to a seated position on the ground, parallel to his head. I still have my scrubs on from the hospital. I didn't have time to change when my mom called.

"Your dad's having a heart attack," she said, before I could even say hello.

"Is he awake, is he talking?" I asked as I tried to assess the situation over the phone. The nurse in me instinctively begins the triage process.

"No," she said, "they are working on him now." I felt a wave of nausea sweep over me. He's not conscious. Six percent. I grabbed my shoes and ran to the car, driving as fast as I could.

Their house is not far from mine, maybe five minutes, but it might as well have been on the other side of the city. Time slows down in these situations. You notice minute details, and they become burned into your memory. Even now, when I stop at the light near their house, I feel the muscles tighten in my neck and anxiety seems to come from nowhere. Why is it that some memories are so vividly recalled, while others slip away unnoticed? We know from research that this is mostly chemical in nature and a response to stress. Humans remember emotional events better than neutral ones. The reason this occurs is mainly because of actions of the adrenal stress hormones. Epinephrine, norepinephrine, and others act on the brain structures responsible for memory.[6] These chemicals help us "lock in" memories for recall at a later time, sometimes to our detriment. During a stressful event, the emotional center of our brain -- the amygdala -- upregulates the nearby hippocampus, allowing it to form a more detailed and stronger memory. The story and emotion involved in the event gives us the ability to recall it later in vivid detail. This recording, etched in our mind, forms a perfect picture of the event, even if the picture we remember is far from perfect. When the memories are traumatic, this "locking in" can result in PTSD.

They finally establish a heartbeat, and they load him in the ambulance. They turn and ask us what hospital we want him taken to.

Someone says, "Can he make it to the Heart Hospital?"

"No, he's not stable enough," they shoot back. We need to go to the nearest hospital.

"Then why did you ask?" I think to myself. There is very little discussion. They load him into the ambulance and close the doors, first one and then the other. It's a sound I've heard hundreds of times—but this time, it sounds so final. Jason, the paramedic and our childhood friend, climbs in with him and they pull away.

In the coming days and months, I would grapple with the decision of taking him to the nearest hospital instead of attempting a higher level of care further away. The "what ifs" would wake me up at night and insert themselves at random times during the day. I would feel guilt— so much guilt—for not demanding we try to make it to a better hospital. I would second guess every action and interaction from those twenty-four hours. I didn't know what story to tell myself, so I painted myself the villain. That's what we do when we don't know what to do, isn't it? We construct a narrative, and it's almost never right. Still…the questions descended on me like mosquitos on a warm summer night. I could barely slap one away before another would come. Did I let him down? Did I play some role in his ultimate demise? Would it have changed the outcome if I had insisted he be taken to another location? What if they had taken him to another hospital and he had died on the way? How would I have lived with that outcome? These questions will forever remain in the realm of conjecture. No real answers, but I would battle the feeling of uncertainty, regret, and profound sadness. The story I told myself took on a life of its own, and I continued to construct a narrative, fueled by grief.

In retrospect, I know it was a desperate attempt to control the situation and somehow alter the outcome. A futile effort at history reconstruction. In the end, all possible roads lead to the same place, but I trace back over the events, searching for that one detail that would render a different result. There is refuge in denial. It's the mind's way of protecting us until the reality of the situation can be fully absorbed. An abstract, psychological process of taking baby steps.

As they take him away, I whisper to my nephew, more as a statement rather than a question, "We're going to have to decide when to turn the ventilator off, aren't we?"

He never turns to look at me; he just nods and says, "Probably." My dad would never fully regain consciousness and would die twenty-four hours later. But our work—the work of grief—was just beginning.

In the book "Option B," Sheryl Sandberg says grief is a demanding companion.[7] In the coming days and weeks, I would come to fully identify with that statement, and many times, I was sure this companion would get the best of me and there would be nothing left.

I turn to go back to my car, and I notice the broken slat on the fence. That board would become symbolic for me. In the next few days, my daughter and son- in-law would replace it with a new board, but the newness of the wood against the weathered slats that flanked either side would be a stark reminder that this was the place where everything changed, a painful reminder that a permanent part of my life no longer existed.

CHAPTER TWO

LISTEN TO THE DYING

Historically, Elisabeth Kübler- Ross has been widely believed to be the authority on grief. I have referenced her theory many times to nursing students in the context of patient and family care. I returned to her writing in the days and weeks that followed Dad's death with a renewed sense of interest in what she had to say. I was seeking her wisdom, not as a teacher, but as someone who needed to understand on a personal level. The first thing that got my attention was this statement: "Listen to the dying. They will tell you everything you need to know about when they are dying. And it's easy to miss."[8] I knew it that summer before he died. My denial was almost too loud to allow me to hear, but that gnawing feeling persisted and so did the uneasiness that made itself at home in the pit of my stomach. Was I the only one who noticed? If so, why?

I tried to brush aside the intrusive thoughts but made it a point to call him for no particular reason and to stop by whenever I passed his office, knowing it would be hard to get away once I was there. He would talk to anyone about anything, and I wanted to talk to him. I desperately tried to arrange a family picture that summer. It was fraught with difficulties from the beginning. Differing schedules, resistance, even an unexpected hospital visit for my dad on the day of one preselected date. It seemed important to me, and I had a sense of urgency. We finally had a date on the calendar, but in the end, that date would coincide with Dad's death. Despite all our efforts, no picture.

So many subtle clues that summer hinted that something was changing. I still look back and wonder, what exactly did I sense? What were the signs that even now, in retrospect, are not clear? A few weeks prior to his death, I attended the funeral of a family friend with my parents. After the service was over and we were leaving, Dad went to step off the curb and I reached to touch his shoulder as I stepped off behind him. At the time, I was struck by how much his shoulder felt like his dad's—my grandfather's—shortly before his death. Was I feeling frailty? Did he seem unsteady? It disturbed me at the time, but I tucked it away and tried to forget the uneasiness I felt.

There were so many vague clues the day was approaching, which in retrospect are more readily aligned with events than they were as it played out in front of my eyes. Isn't that always the way it is? We see clearly looking back in time in a way that's not possible without that perspective. "Listen to the dying." Did he know? Did I? Maybe what I sensed was fear. My fear of losing him was overwhelming at times, and it became harder to ignore. As the warm summer wind began to cool and leaves began to fall, my worry became more focused. Nothing felt right that summer.

During the final hot days of August, when the kids were going back to school, I thought about a book I listened to on tape as a child. When we were young, my mom would check these books out from the library for my sisters and me to listen to as we went to sleep. Our favorite by far was a book by Elizabeth Enright called "Thimble Summer."[9] The story centers around a nine-year-old girl named Garnet. It takes place in the Depression, during a drought that threatens to ruin her family financially. Throughout the book, Garnet is concerned about her dad and the stress he faces as he tries to provide for their family. In the book, the summer is long and hot, and she spends most of it worrying. Eventually, she finds a silver thimble in a dried-up riverbed. The day she finds the thimble, the rain comes. On the tape, you can hear the rain hitting the metal roof, slowly at first, then coming down hard. Garnet thinks the thimble is magic. I always loved this part of the story. I thought about that silver thimble a lot that August before Dad died, and about a time in my life when I would drift off to sleep to the sound of the narrator's voice, confident in how the story would end. I wished the ending to this story would be magic as well. But deep inside...I knew the ending would come too soon and the story would be anything but magical.

I now know I was experiencing anticipatory grief. Anticipatory grief is the beginning of the end in our minds, and it occurs while we still operate in two distinct worlds, one that we know and one that is unsafe, where someone we love no longer exists. In this kind of grief, we are focused on the loss ahead. It is a sort of double grief.[10] People often experience this when someone close to them is dying and the outcome is certain, but the course is slow. Maybe I needed more time to adjust to the loss. Maybe I just worried more than the average person.

When we were young, my parents decided (mostly my mom) that if they were ever going to get ahead, my dad would need to go back to school. So, in the fall of 1974, he moved to Stillwater, a town in Northeastern Oklahoma. He would come home for church on Wednesday nights and drive back to school on Thursday mornings. Every Friday after class, he would drive home for the weekend and leave again the following Monday morning. At night, when he was gone, we got to talk to him before bed. Because it was long distance and because money was tight, our calls were timed by an hourglass that sat next to the phone. Each turn of the hourglass represented one minute, and we each got two minutes. While I talked, I watched the sand slowly slip from the top of the hourglass to the bottom. I don't remember much about those conversations—nothing really, in fact—but I do remember watching the sand and worrying that it would soon be gone from the top of the hourglass and my time with him would be over. I was fearful, even as a small child, and those phone calls were reassuring to me. I hadn't thought about that hourglass in years, but as my dad lay dying, it was one of the first things I thought about, and I wondered how much sand was left in the top of the hourglass, how much had already fallen to the bottom.

After losing his wife, C.S. Lewis began the arduous task of grieving. In his book "A Grief Observed," he says, "No one ever told me that grief felt so much like fear. I am not afraid, but the sensation is like being afraid. The same fluttering in the stomach, the same restlessness, the yawning."[11] Unlike Lewis, I did feel afraid, but afraid of what? Afraid of my life without him, of forgetting his voice? Afraid of my own mortality? Maybe just afraid. The fear I felt was surprising, but the anger I felt after his death was shocking. Even though I knew it was one of the predictable stages of grief, it still caught me off guard.

Kübler-Ross says there are five stages to grief. These stages are:

- Denial – This is most often the first stage of grief, and it is necessary to help people survive the loss. Many experience shock and disbelief, or report feeling numb. Denial is nature's way of only letting in as much as can be handled in the moment. As denial fades, they are better able to cope with the emotions that are suppressed in the very early stages.

- Anger – People who grieve will often go through this stage, but one thing to remember is that anger is often a cover for many other emotions. Generally, they will get to these different emotions in time, but it's important to understand this stage is normal and important to healing.

- Bargaining – In this stage, people often bargain with God for more time, for healing, or to somehow rid themselves of the pain. It's the mind's way to negotiate our way out of hurt.

- Depression – This stage is a natural response to loss and comes with the realization that someone they love will no longer be a part of their physical environment. It can feel like this stage will last forever, but it is actually an important part of the healing process.

- Acceptance – In this stage, people come to terms with the loss. It doesn't mean they won't wish it were different, but they stop fighting with reality and look for a new normal.

These stages are not linear; rather, they are navigated in an individualistic pattern that often repeats. Patients may get stuck in one stage or another before briefly moving on and revisiting the same stage again. After my dad's death, I distinctly remember being in a store and seeing an older person shopping. They looked much older than Dad had been when he died. It made me angry. Why were they still here, alive, shopping in Walmart, and my dad was dead? This directional anger at perfect strangers caught me off guard. The injustice of it all fueled my discontent and kept me stirred up inside. So much anger. Sometimes, when a person is grieving, this anger is directed toward others or the person who died. This can cause significant distress for the person who is mourning. They may be angry for a variety of reasons, maybe because the person didn't seek medical attention soon enough, didn't wear a seatbelt, or died by suicide. They may be angry at themselves for their perceived role in the death. Understanding the anger and moving past it may take professional help, but in most situations, it will take time to put the death and resulting emotions in perspective.

While Kübler-Ross's grief theory is a valid way to categorize a grief pathway, newer research has constructed a different framework. After Freud's *Mourning and Melancholia,* there were seven decades of general consensus by psychologists and psychiatrists that to successfully navigate grief, the mourner would need to disengage from the deceased. According to this accepted belief, any continued attachment would signal a dysfunctional grief and would be viewed as abnormal. Even Freud, in writing to a friend whose daughter had just died, confessed that after nine long years, his grief for his own daughter remained unconsoled. He struggled, but the answers never came, and the void was never filled. His grief remained painful for many years. As time would pass, a more contemporary discourse about grief would begin to take place.[12] The new approach would be labeled "Continuing Bonds."

In the continuing bonds model, instead of "moving on," a phrase that tends to rub people the wrong way, the grieving person finds ways to redefine the relationship. Continuing ties to the loved one can be healthy and beneficial as the bereaved person learns to live in the new environment without the person they lost. Instead of relinquishing the bond, they retain it.

The purpose of grief is...the construction of a durable biography that enables the living to integrate the memory of the dead into their ongoing lives; the process by which this is achieved is principally conversation with others who knew the deceased.[13]

The term continuing bonds was originally coined from child-development studies relating to parental attachment. This attachment is why grief is so hard. We are attached to the person we lost, and just because that person dies, it doesn't mean the attachment is gone. So, finding a way to maintain that attachment is paramount to healthy grieving. This is a completely different direction from what we previously thought. My attachment to my dad was so strong, so important, I grieved not only his physical loss, but also my emotional attachment to him as well. This continuing bond with him is a further manifestation of that secure attachment. Finding ways to maintain the relationship in a new context is a continuing bond at its best, and it can ease the transition from the physical presence of our loved one to a metaphysical one. This new relationship, like the one when our loved one was living, is not static but rather dynamic and changing. No longer are relationships limited to those of reciprocity only between the living. Continuing bonds are important if we are to navigate our losses. Continuing that attachment is a healthy way to move through grief. I was thankful my research showed me this and encouraged me to continue that bond, albeit in a different way, with my dad. His physical absence didn't have to mean my relationship with him was over, just that it had changed.

CHAPTER THREE

THE ROOM

In the emergency department (ED), we wait. They put us in a small room off to the side. Unless you work there or have had a loved one in critical condition, you probably wouldn't even know it was there or the purpose for the space. There are two long sofa-like benches and a couple of chairs. The whole room has a sparse feel, like maybe the furniture has been there from the sixties. If there were windows in that room, I don't remember them. There are tissues in boxes at the end of each sofa. You know, the kind of tissue that falls apart when it's used? Fragile, one-ply tissues, unable to withstand any pressure put on them. I looked at those boxes, and in that moment, I identified with the tissue. Fragile, ready to fall apart. I've passed this room hundreds of times when I've worked in this department in the past. Even now, a year later,

I avoid that room. It's a small space, but I feel it could swallow me whole if I get too near. So much bad news is delivered in this room. The floors are stained with thousands of tears. Families often exit this room into a different world, one that is unfamiliar and forever changed.

Our family is large, and we spill out into the hall. No one comes to update us. We wait. I grow impatient and go to find someone to get a report. An ED physician comes back with me and tells us Dad is stable and they are taking him to the Cath Lab. "His vital signs look good," he says, "and his pupils are reactive." I know this means he still has some brain function, but how much? What is the scope of damage? He takes us to another area where there is more room and our family can be together. It's right outside the procedure room. It's torture, and the minutes creep by. More friends fill the room and we wait.

After some time, the interventional cardiologist emerges. I don't know him. He seems agitated, and I immediately take a dislike to him. "I need two decision makers to step forward and only two," he says in a demanding voice. My mind flashes back to the movie *The Hunger Games*. We all look at each other. Two of us step forward and the others stay within earshot.

"I just need to know if you want me to do chest compressions, because it's not going to matter," he says with his body turned away from us.

Not going to matter? Not going to matter to who? Because it matters to us. We surround him and begin asking him what he has tried. We are not without experience and what we are asking is reasonable.

He looks irritated, annoyed that we are asking questions. "Look," he says, with one hand on his hip. "He's in complete pump failure; he's not going to make it." I remember thinking he sounded like he was just telling us about a car. "Engine's shot; get a new car."

My niece says, "I'm having a problem with your attitude." He just stares at us, but his body posture softens a bit. The full reality of what we are facing comes into sharp focus, and we look at each other. Realization begins to settle on us like a heavy, wet blanket and we feel the weight of the truth as it is forced on us. "Would you like to see him before we take him to ICU?" he says.

We move slowly toward the procedure room. He is on a ventilator and the monitor makes a familiar sound, although everything seems foreign to me. He is laying there in a hospital gown. He doesn't have a blanket on, and I think he must be cold even though subconsciously I know he is unaware. There are others in the room, but in my memory, they seem like shadowy figures, almost like the lens of a camera has blurred the picture to only focus on my dad. We approach him: me, my mom, and my three sisters. He doesn't move. We spend a few minutes with him in this room then kiss him and tell him we love him. My footsteps feel heavy as we walk away. My body feels strange, like the legs that are supporting me belong to someone else. I struggle to reconnect my head with the parts of my body that suddenly seem foreign. If someone had told me I was floating, I would have believed them.

The interaction with this physician will forever change the way I approach families in crisis. As healthcare providers, it's important to begin healing at the point of trauma, and part of that process is being aware of our body language and words. Kindness in these situations can help the family cope. It is important to their long-term recovery. Often, healthcare workers seem emotionally detached from the situation. That can come across to the family as uncaring. Part of this response from the healthcare staff is protective. They are witness to this kind of trauma every single day. I know this from my own experiences with patients and their families. It wears on you; over time, it wears you down. At some point, we detach, but the resulting complication can be further trauma to the family.

During my dad's short hospital stay prior to his death, we also encountered kind nurses and doctors. They were gentle with us, gave us their undivided attention, and helped us make those hard, end-of-life decisions. I will forever be grateful to a nurse named Dana, who patiently dealt with the eight nurses in our family. She helped begin our healing prior to Dad's death. Nurses have a difficult job. We not only have to be experts in our fields, we must care for families in crisis. It is a physically and emotionally demanding job. There have been many times in my career when I have held it together at the bedside, only to cry all the way home. These deaths add up over time, and the weight can be suffocating. I am grateful we had someone to walk with us during that twenty-four hours. I ask healthcare providers—the ones I teach and the ones with whom I practice—to understand the concept of caring for these families. In being proactive, we are practicing preventive medicine. Our actions, when delivered in a caring way, can lay the foundation for optimal healing. Even when the news is bad, compassion can ease the message.

Without careful consideration of our communication, long-term depression, dysfunctional grief, and PTSD can be the result. At that moment, when the physician said, "It's not going to matter," we lost faith in him. We didn't believe he had our dad's best interest at heart, and it caused us to doubt that Dad was given the best chance for survival. This five-minute interaction would complicate our grief in the days ahead.

After we leave Dad's side, we join the rest of our family and friends. I don't remember going upstairs to the ICU, but I vaguely remember saying I knew the way. I am familiar with this hospital; it must be instinct taking over as we wind down halls and load onto an elevator. We make it to the second floor before my dad gets there. We stand in the hall just outside the elevator. No one says a word. There are people around me, but I am almost unaware. I stare at the elevator. The bell rings, the doors open, and I see my dad. He is accompanied by two nurses. He is intubated and does not move. At some point, he has vomited blood. Was it the rough intubation? Is he bleeding internally? Again, I triage. They tell us to wait until they get him settled.

I stare out the window into the dark night. I'm thinking about when I was a child, maybe five or six. One night, I heard something outside and saw a flashing light. I was frightened and called to my dad. He came into my room, and I crawled out of bed. He looked out the window as I cowered behind him. This seemed to be a standard position for us. Him in front, me hiding behind him. There was something going on at the house behind us. He told me to go back to bed and not to worry, it was nothing. I was struck by the irony that this time, on this dark night, the thing to fear was inside, where it was light. It's strange what you think about when your world is changing so rapidly.

In his book, "The Orphaned Adult," Alexander Levy says, "There is no experience quite as stunning as when there is nothing where something has always been."[14] This is somewhat like Piaget's object permanence theory. Babies in sensorimotor stage do not understand that when you hide a ball under a blanket, the ball still exists. Once the baby enters the preoperational stage, they understand the concept that the ball still exists somewhere, even if it disappears. They look for it. I think this is one reason death is so difficult to wrap our heads around. From the time we master object permanence as a baby, we look for things that go away. Accepting the fact that the person we loved will never return goes against everything we have learned. Like the baby playing a game, we keep looking, albeit subconsciously, for the object of our desire to come back. Object permeance is a powerful premise to overcome when death is the cause for the absence. For those who believe in God, as I do, faith is what we substitute for the missing object: "the substance of things hoped for, evidence of things not seen" (Heb. 11:1).

I know he is slipping away. We all do. Any hope we had for his recovery is fading with every hour that passes. How could this be? How could my dad not exist anymore? The death of a parent is especially difficult. Levy goes on to say, "Parents play an entirely unique role: Whatever else can be said about them, they are the first and the most prominent continuous certainty in our lives. We are aware of them before we become aware of anything else. We have gotten used to them before we even learn of life's other constants like the sun, the moon, or the ground."[15] Levy was right. My constant wasn't constant anymore.

One evening, sometime after my dad died, my husband and I were sitting in our library at home, he in his recliner, and I in mine. This room in our house is filled with books from ceiling to floor. There is a rolling library ladder on one wall whose main purpose, I have decided, is for kids to climb up and jump off. He loves this room. I, on the other hand, think it smells like an old library. Like a place where lots of old books are stored. On this night, he was reading a book and I was worrying. This was our usual activity. "I don't think I will ever get over my dad's death," I said. There was a long pause. He didn't even look up from the book he was reading but began quoting a passage from Shakespeare's *Hamlet* where Claudius is imploring a depressed Hamlet to emerge from his sadness after his father's death. Claudius begins his speech saying,

Tis sweet and commendable in your nature, Hamlet,

To give these mourning duties to your father.

But you must know your father lost a father,

That father lost, lost his, and the survivor bound

In filial obligation for some term

To do obsequious sorrow.[16]

I stared blankly at him. "Everyone loses their father at some point, honey," he further clarified. I must have looked confused. "It's the way the world works," he added and sounded both sympathetic and somehow authoritative at the same time.

"Yeah," I said, resuming my worry, "but Hamlet didn't lose *my* dad, did he?"

He closed his book, laid it in his lap, and looked over at me, "No, babe, Hamlet didn't lose your dad. And you're right—it's different," he said. And I knew he meant it.

When people go through grief, they often feel isolated, and intellectually knowing that death is a common—even expected—outcome does little to comfort them. It can feel lonely and foreign, like traveling alone to a place you've never been. The way feels long when you are by yourself and don't know where you are going. All the familiar landmarks that logged your progress have somehow disappeared. That's how grief feels. It reminds me of when I am trying to follow Siri's directions in the car, but I keep making a wrong turn and she keeps saying, "Redirecting, proceed to the route." And I keep thinking, "I don't know what route I'm supposed to take. Do I even know where the destination is? And if I don't, how in the world will I know when I have reached it?" No matter what your loss, grief is a lonely journey.

There comes a point in everyone's life where, like Hamlet, we lose our fathers. For some, that loss is complicated by conflicting feelings. Not all parent-child relationships are healthy; not all are therapeutic. The size of the hole left in our lives will differ based on these past experiences. But for me, the loss of my dad left a crater so wide and so deep that, often, I felt I might fall over the edge into the hole where he disappeared. Time passes. Things change. The hole remains.

CHAPTER FOUR

FEAR

I slip into the ICU where he is being cared for. We take turns sitting with him. Generally, when patients are in critical care, the hospital allows only two family members at the bedside, but they are more lenient with us. Sometimes, there are three or four of us in the room, maybe because they know we will stay out of the way, or maybe because they know he is dying. We have all, the nurses in our family, been on the other side of this equation before. Having to deal with families like us. Part of me feels sorry for these nurses and doctors, trying to do their work under our scrutiny.

I am familiar with these sights and sounds. I see a former student coming out of his room, and I wonder, "Does he know enough to be here doing this?" I want somebody with experience. I stare at Dad, but he doesn't move. He is sedated by the drugs they have given him, so he can rest and to keep him from fighting the ventilator. I sit in the chair next to his bed. They have cleaned him up. The blood on his gown is gone, and he seems peaceful.

His ring finger is bandaged. When patients are in ICU, they can begin to swell from the fluids we give them. Taking their rings off early is important to prevent them from having to be cut off. We almost waited too late for my dad. Earlier in the night, my nephew, Jason, asked if anyone had dental floss. He wanted to use it to wrap around my dad's finger to make the diameter smaller, so the ring would slip off. I looked in my purse; I knew I had some. I have everything in my purse. I pulled out a package of the floss and handed it over. They all stared at me. My purse has always been a joke. I thought to myself, "I need to be on that TV game show 'Let's Make a Deal.'" They have a segment where the host asks contestants to pull a requested object out of their bag. If they have it, they win money. I would be good at that game. When we finally got his wedding ring off, it tore the skin where his ring had been. It seems strange and painful to see gauze around his finger where his ring should be. I don't think I ever saw him without it. I think about the dental floss. When I originally put it in my purse, it never crossed my mind that I would use it to remove my dad's wedding ring from his finger.

But I did a lot of things that night I never thought I would have to do.

We are in the first twenty-four hours after his collapse. He seems stable for now, but I know that doesn't mean anything. How many times have I said to patient families, "We won't know anything for twenty-four hours"? Patients are often stable during this window, but then multiple organ failure begins. They are stable until they are not, and then it all falls apart quickly. There are many times during this process that I find myself wishing I didn't know what would happen. In a strange way, I envy those who are clueless about these things. If I knew less, I could maintain some sort of hope… But I know too much to hope. . . I already know how this story will end, and unlike the book on tape I listened to as a child, there is no pause button I can press to stop the story from progressing. There is no magic thimble and no saving rain hitting the roof. This story will end no matter what I do, or what I wish.

I listen to the rhythmic sounds of the machine, effortlessly doing for him what he can no longer do for himself. He has been lulled into a drug-induced coma where his life will end with the slow drip of an IV. I reach for his hand; I'm thinking about being nine years old again. We are riding bikes. Most Sundays after church he would take me and my older sister, Cindy, riding while my mom put our two little sisters down for a nap. We had those banana-seat bikes with the big handlebars that were so popular in the seventies. I loved that bike and the pink streamers that hung from the plastic grips. On this particular day, in my memory, it is only Dad and me, and we are riding down a gravel road. It's rough and I feel uncertain of my balance on the shifting rocks, so I am already a little apprehensive. We come to a large grate in the road and he rides over it, but I stop just short.

He turns to look for me and rides back. "What's wrong?" he says.

"I'm scared," I reply.

"Scared of what?" he asks, looking around for the perceived threat I am referencing.

"I'm scared of falling into that hole," I say as I peer over the edge. It is deep and dark, and I see my reflection in the muddy water. I begin to imagine the things that might be lurking just under the surface, ready to grab a little girl and pull her under. I back up even further, just to be safe.

He rides back over the grate in an effort to prove it will hold up under my weight. "Come on," he says, "you won't fall, I promise." I am not convinced. He gets off his bike and walks over to the grate and begins jumping up and down. My heart is pounding, and I worry he will fall through the grate into oblivion and I will never see him again. I feel a wave of nausea and my knees go weak.

"Let's just go home," I plead, as I turn my bike around.

"We're not going home," he says. "You can't spend the rest of your life avoiding grates."

"Watch me," I say defiantly. He walks back to me, takes hold of the handlebars of my bike, and begins to pull me over the grate. I dig my heels in, dragging gravel to the edge as I hear it hit the water with a splash. He continues pulling as if he doesn't even notice my resistance. We reach the other side, and to my surprise, we don't plunge into the darkness.

"I told you it was safe," he says matter-of -factly as he gets back on his bike.

We ride down the road with the wind in our hair. The anxiety completely melts away. My shoes are covered in gravel dust from the failed resistance, but I feel brave. I feel strong. When I get back home, I will tell Cindy all about it, but I will leave out the part where Dad pulls me over the grate. "She doesn't need to know everything," I think to myself. How could I have been so afraid of a stupid grate? It seems silly now that I am safely on the other side.

The IV machine begins to beep, and I instinctively reach to silence it, check the bag of fluid, and press the call button for the nurse. "This seems like a grate all over again," I think as I stare at his hand resting motionlessly on the bed, but I can't tell which side he is on. There is no sun on our faces, no wind in our hair, but the fear is very much the same. Only this time, I'm not nine and this time he won't come back for me. I stare at my dad. So many of my memories are wrapped up in him. So many things only *we* know. Who will remember these things with me? When I don't have my facts straight, who will help me sort them out? Who will pull me over the grate and prove to me once again the world is a safe place? He is the keeper of so much, and I wonder: how much has already been lost?

I think about my purse again and all the things I put in it to be prepared "just in case". There's nothing in my purse that can fix this, and I think about Mary Poppins and her magic carpet bag. Even Mary, who is practically perfect in every way, couldn't have prepared for this. I slip out of the ICU and back into the waiting room. My dad hated hospitals. I think I do, too, which is unfortunate since it's what I do for a living.

CHAPTER FIVE

THE NIGHT IS LONG

We spend the night in the waiting room, leaning against each other for support, both emotionally and physically. The night is long and the chairs, not made for sleeping, offer little comfort. We take turns sitting with my dad in the ICU. There is little change in his condition. When it's my time to sit with him, I check his urinary catheter bag hanging on the side of the bed. He is still making some urine. This is a good sign. It means he hasn't suffered total kidney damage, and they are still working on some level. I spend a lot of my time at his side, looking for hope in any place I can find it but knowing deep down inside, in the end, it's not going to matter. Still I look. Still I hope, because hope is gentler than no hope.

Occasionally, someone else's family member wanders into the waiting room that we have commandeered. We must all give them a subliminal signal to go away because they look around the room and turn and leave. Just as well, I think. I don't feel much like small talk with strangers, and we had pretty much filled the room with our family anyway. We stay this way for hours, sleeping intermittently.

My mom spends most of the night in a chair by his bed with her head resting on the mattress where he sleeps. This will be the last night they spend together. They have been married for fifty-five years and together since she was fifteen and he was eighteen. It will all come to an end in this room. I think back to my wedding day and wonder: "Will my marriage end this way, someday?" In retrospect, we are grateful for these twenty-four hours. Grateful his life didn't end in the driveway. Thankful we had a few precious hours to wrap our heads around what was taking place. Our family wanders in and out of the ICU, alternating between the waiting room and his bed. None of us hold out much hope that his situation will improve. We know too much, but even with this knowledge, there is a powerful desire to believe he will wake up. We have all—the nurses in our family—been witness to miracles. Patients who should have never walked out of the hospital, babies who should have never survived and yet—they do. Where is our miracle? Why won't we be granted this mercy? I know there is no real answer to this question—still I ask, still I wonder.

As the sun begins to come up over the horizon and fill the room like liquid spilling over everything, my sister Chris and I decide to go back to my house to change clothes and brush our teeth. When we get there, my family is still sleeping. My sister decides to lie down on the couch and rest for a few minutes. I slip into the bathroom and turn on the shower. I never take a shower, always a bath, but for some reason I reach for the handle and turn the water to hot. I slip out of my clothes and step in. As the water begins to stream down my body, I begin to cry. The noise of the water obliterates the sound of sadness that pours out of me like a river that has broken its levee. I lean against the shower wall for support and let the tears fall, mixing with the water as they mingle and rush down the drain. I don't know how long I stand there crying, but my throat begins to ache, and the bathroom fills with steam. Strange thoughts are running through my head. Maybe if I don't go back to the hospital, he won't die. Maybe I dreamed the whole thing. Maybe he will be awake, sitting up in bed when I return. I put my hands over my face and press hard as if the pressure will slow the irrational thoughts. This magical thinking has no bearing on reality. I know this—but the thoughts still come.

I shut the water off and grab a towel. I feel exhausted, but I'm not sure if it's from sleeping in a chair all night, the confusion I feel, or the situation. It is probably a combination of all these things. I quickly get dressed and wake my sister. We head back to the hospital.

They have decided to try and bring my dad out of the drug-induced coma he has been in since he was brought to the hospital, so we can better assess the damage. At some point, he opens his eyes. I am on one side of the bed, and my mom is on the other.

"Dad," I say. He looks over at me. He has a strange look on his face, an expression I have never seen. Is it confusion or fear?

"Jim," my mom says, and he looks at her. Is this a response? Is he cognitive?

I wish I could remember what happened next. I have no further recollection of this part of the experience. For some reason, it is blocked from my memory. Why didn't I ask him to blink if he could understand me? Why didn't I try to get him to squeeze my hand if he could process what I was saying? We do this with patients all the time. Why did I not do this with him? The nurse in me dissolved into the daughter, and my training seemed to fall away. Was his response just a reflex? Was his movement meaningful? At some point, his heart rate goes too high, and he must be sedated again. Why didn't I tell him not to be afraid? How many times had he done that for me? His eyes still haunt me, and I wonder, "Did he know? Did he understand what was happening?" I worried about this for some time after his death. Later, my niece would tell me that she did test his cognitive ability. There was no meaningful response.

By the evening, twenty-three hours after his collapse, things begin to go downhill quickly. His heart rate becomes erratic; his blood pressure begins to fall. He is dying. We have been asking for a cardiologist, but whether they haven't contacted him, or he chooses not to come is unclear to me at this point. A hospitalist comes in to see him. They have my dad on what we call "pressors." This is a category of medications to keep his blood pressure up. The physician offers to have him sent to another hospital where he can be placed on extracorporeal membrane oxygenation (ECMO). ECMO is a machine that takes blood from the body, oxygenates it using an artificial lung, and pumps it back into the body using an artificial heart. We discuss this with each other and our family friend and pediatrician, Dr. Harmon. My mom is standing with us.

"Help me make this decision," she says. We look at each other and collectively shake our heads no.

My sister Cindy says, "He may die on the way to the other hospital, and I don't want him to die alone."

We know we are prolonging the inevitable. We step back into the room. My brother-in-law Mike, who is a nurse practitioner, asks them to shut off the pressors. The slow drip of the IV comes to a halt, and the ventilator stops. He ceases to exist. My dad would transition from this life to the next to the soft sound of us singing "Amazing Grace."

One by one we leave his bedside. There is nothing left for us to do. As we are leaving the room, someone hands us a white, opaque, plastic bag with my dad's things in it. Inside is the last shirt he wore, the pants that were cut at the scene, his belt, and his undershirt. The bag says, "patient belongings," but he's not a patient anymore so I wonder, "Who do his belongings belong to?" My mom says she doesn't want to see the bag. I don't either. My sister Cindy takes it; we never discuss it again. To this day, I don't know what happened to that bag. Sometime later, I would hand a bag just like it to one of my patient's family members, and I would remember *that* night, *that* bag, *that* pain. I would choke back tears that seemed to rise from my chest like heat off an asphalt road in the summer.

Grief can be unpredictable that way, surprising us when we least expect it. We face our loss in a hundred different ways on a hundred different days and it's hard to anticipate when or where the next attack will come. We are always unprepared for the ambush. The sounds of that night would fill my head: the beeping IV, the muffled cries, the regular rush of air through the ventilator finally replaced by a deep and deafening silence. Grief is noisy, isn't it? It will be heard above everything else and will demand our attention, even when we try to ignore it. Sometimes that noise will come from a simple, white, plastic bag.

CHAPTER SIX

THE UNPLANNED GOODBYE

Soon after my dad is pronounced dead, we slip out of the SICU and go back to the waiting room. We begin to gather our things and move the furniture back to its original position. Even in grief, we are an orderly bunch. I pull my mom aside and ask her about the funeral home where they have made their arrangements. My mom is a planner, and she had taken care of this a few years prior. She made me store the urns in my attic because she said Dad didn't want them in theirs. She tells me the name of the funeral home. I say, "I think that's where Kim works."

The summer before I got engaged to my husband, I spent a lot of time with a guy I met while selling children's shoes at a department store. I worked there through high school and college. Mike worked in the men's shoe department at the same store. We spent that summer together mainly wasting time and having fun. That next year, I would go on to marry my husband, and later, Mike would marry Kim. Our paths would not cross very often, and it had been at least ten years since I had seen either one of them.

I quickly message her and tell her about my dad's death and that we are at the hospital. She sends a message back that she does indeed work for the funeral home where my mom had made their arrangements and she will take care of everything. I am suddenly filled with relief. What a blessing that my relationship with Mike, so long ago, would bring Kim into my life at such a traumatic time. That God saw a need that wouldn't happen for another thirty-seven years, and he laid the groundwork for it to be met so far in advance. He was preparing for the pain I didn't even know I would experience. What a comfort it was to me to be able to call her and let her help our family. When we had to leave the hospital and my dad's body behind, I knew she would make sure he was cared for. Kim made the arduous task of beginning to let go a little easier that night. She took control when we were so blinded by grief we didn't know where to turn. My two nieces and nephew stayed with my dad as they prepared his body for transfer to the funeral home. They are all nurses, and it was one last, final gift they gave to him, and us.

That night, my sisters and I stayed with my mom at her house. I slipped into a bed in the guest bedroom and lay there. I was physically and emotionally exhausted but determined to stay awake until midnight. I wanted to soak up every minute of the last day I had a dad. I watched the clock until it read 12:00. At some point after that, I drifted off into a fitful sleep.

We were scheduled to meet Kim the next day at the funeral home. My mom, sisters, and I arrive the next afternoon to make the arrangements. I can't even begin to tell you how much gratitude I feel when I see Kim's face. Just to have someone I know somehow makes me feel better. She leads us into her office. There is paperwork to fill out, and someone has to sign the informant line on the death certificate. Somehow, it ends up in my hands. I don't think anyone wants to sign it. I stare at the page. Finally, I write the date of his death where it is requested, 11/17/17. I'm still shocked by this. I sign my name and list daughter under relationship. I quickly hand the clipboard back to Kim as if getting it out of my possession will make me feel better. It doesn't. It won't be the last time I struggle with writing down the date of his death.

A few months after Dad died, I went to see a new doctor. They handed me a clipboard and asked me to fill out some background history, current issues, etc. I didn't think anything about it. I was reading through the questions—what medications are you on, have you been hospitalized in the last year, what is your complaint today—and then I come to it. Family history, father's health: excellent, good, fair, poor, or **DEAD**. The word dead was not really in all caps or bolded, but it might as well have been. I suddenly forgot how to breathe. I was frozen. I stared at the paper. I didn't want to put a check mark under the word "dead." It caught me completely off guard and tears suddenly filled my eyes and spilled over my lower lids. I couldn't see anything. Everything was blurry as I tried to see through the water that had flooded my eyes. I was a complete mess. I forced myself to breathe and discreetly tried to wipe the tears away that seemed to be coming from an open faucet. My chest felt tight, and my throat seemed to be closing off.

I stood up, grabbed my purse, and took the paperwork to the bathroom with me. Inside the safety of the bathroom, I cry—or rather sob. There's no place to sit, so I sit on the toilet to finish filling out the forms. "This is ridiculous," I thought to myself.

I could just hear Dad, "Let me get this straight—you got up from a perfectly good chair to sit on a toilet in a dirty bathroom, so you can put a checkmark in a box?" "Yeah, Dad," I said out loud. "I did, and it's all your fault." It made me feel better to blame him for my weakness. I finished the paperwork and exited the stall. I caught a glimpse of myself in the bathroom mirror and moved closer to fix my make up because I might have been sad, but I refused to be sad *and* ugly. I walked back to the office and handed the clipboard to the receptionist, acting like *everybody* sits on the toilet to fill out paperwork. This sudden sadness would constantly surprise me. That's how I would continue to feel for months, never knowing when some innocent mention of death would send me off or set me back.

At the funeral home, Kim goes over the plans for the service and makes suggestions. He will be cremated. Thank God we don't have to pick out a casket. I think that might have pushed me over the edge. I had been over the edge so often by that point, I thought of listing it as a summer home, like rich people do. They reside in New York, Chicago, and Over the Edge. She gives us several options for memorial items: things they can do with fingerprints, necklaces to put ashes in, urns. Then I notice a candle displayed with the other items. She sees me looking at it. "We can have his picture put on it," she says.

I know she has to offer this to us, but I suddenly have an irresistible urge to burst out laughing. I can just hear my Dad: "So, you're going to cremate me and then make a candle with my picture on it, so my face will glow? I don't think so."

"I'm the absolute worst," I think to myself. I move fluidly between sobbing and making tacky remarks. My dad would be so proud. Mostly of the tacky remarks, not so much the sobbing.

Our family meets that evening to write my dad's obituary. We try the regular format, listing those proceeding him in death and those who he is survived by, but we aren't happy with any of it. I decide to type, "Jim Archer was survived by one beautiful daughter, and three average ones." It just went downhill from there. We started writing it from a funny point of view and knew he would love it. We convinced my mom to let us publish it, but the Daily Oklahoman had other ideas. I guess they didn't share our sense of humor. Below are a couple of segments from the original obituary, prior to their revisions. We published this version online.

On November 17th, the day that Jim Archer passed away, he did not read the morning paper. Normally, Jim liked to start his day by scouring the Daily Oklahoman for any item of interest. It is widely believed that he was the last person on earth to maintain this practice—we fear the Oklahoman may not long survive him.

The previous statement was retracted from the printed version of the obituary at the Daily Oklahoman. They stated that it was not reflective of the opinions of their readers (the three they have left) and they would not print it.

When he had finished his research and notified various parties of his findings, he would turn to the obituary column. "Well," he would announce to anyone who was listening, "my name's not in here today, so I guess I'll go to work." And so he did—generously sharing his talents, time, wisdom, love, and jokes with everyone he met.

Jimmy Darrell Archer was born on September 1, 1942, in Tishomingo, Oklahoma, to Frank A. Archer and Bonnie Mae Potts. After the war, he moved with his parents to Oklahoma City, where he attended Southeast High School, graduating in 1961. At Southeast, he met Judy K. Fanning, who became the love of his life. Together they married, made a home, raised one beautiful daughter, and three average ones......

Details of Dad's life followed, but we ended with this postscript:

P.S. Dad always hated that obituaries didn't list the cause of death. So, in his honor, if you would like to have a detailed account of how he died, send a self-addressed, stamped envelope and $1 to: Jim Archer Homes......... Proceeds will be donated to The Children's Ministry at Bethany First Church of the Nazarene.

The last part of the obituary was only meant as a joke, but the letters and money began to arrive. So, I had to write a detailed account of what happened. He would have loved this so much.

CHAPTER SEVEN

DREAMS OF THE DEAD

I didn't dream about my dad the first few weeks after his death. Surprising, since my every waking thought was about him. Maybe my mind was too exhausted. Maybe I was just protecting myself, but I was strangely troubled by his absence in my dreams. It wasn't until several weeks later he appeared. I dreamed we were at his funeral. The church was big, and there were flowers at the front. His casket was in the center. There were hundreds of people there, but I couldn't make out their faces. They seemed far away. I knew he was still alive, trapped in the casket. I ran to the front of the church and tried to pry the lid open, but it was too heavy. I begged someone to help me, but they just looked at me. No one came to help. I was desperate. I knew he was running out of air. I screamed, but no noise came out of my throat, as if I were paralyzed. I woke with a start and sat straight up in bed, shaking. I lay there for quite some time, afraid to close my eyes. Finally, I slipped out of bed and crept to the living room, huddling there in a chair to stave off the inevitability of sleep, afraid of the story that might unfold if I slipped off again, afraid the paralysis would take control of my body. My dad had returned to me in my dreams, and it was the worst dream I had ever had.

This phenomenon is called sleep paralysis. When it occurs outside of a medical condition, it's called isolated sleep paralysis (ISP). When people experience ISP, vivid hallucinations are common, but the sensorium remains clear. The hallucinatory rapid eye movement (REM) content of sleep paralysis appears to be somewhat different from normal dreaming. We know that 30% of dreams are frightening, but ISP is characterized by fear approximately 90% of the time.[17] This paralysis can be very disturbing. Individuals are asleep but acutely aware they cannot move. It can intensify the fear experienced by the dreamer.

In retrospect, I think this dream was a way for me to work through feelings that I was in some way responsible for his death, that I could have done something to prevent it or could have altered its course once put into motion. He was always so proud of the fact that we were nurses. I had let him down when he had needed me most, something he had never done to me.

I was discussing this guilt I felt with a friend, and he said he felt the same thing after his dad died. He gave permission for the physician to place his dad on a ventilator, something he understood to be the final step before death. Intellectually, he knew he was not responsible for his dad's death, but he viewed this consent as his part in his dad's passing. In caring for patients, I know guilt plays a role in the struggle to come to terms with loss, but hearing him say he felt the same thing I did was somehow comforting and healing, like I wasn't alone in my reaction to the trauma of death. It normalized the emotion for me, and I was grateful for his vulnerability.

It is common for people to dream of their loved ones after their death. Research suggests that 58% of those who have lost a loved one report dreaming of the deceased.[18] Often, those dreams are therapeutic. They can help the bereaved cope with the loss more effectively and provide a space to remain connected.[19] However, in some studies, there is compelling evidence that the traumatic event is sometimes partially reexperienced as a nightmare.[20] This can be disturbing to the individual and can begin a cycle of insomnia, signaling dysfunctional grief. When these dreams persist, professional help may be indicated.

I dreamed about my dad only one other time in that first year. It wasn't the same dream, but it was equally unpleasant. I decided if I never dreamed about my dad again, it would be fine by me. For some, dreams about a loved one can be therapeutic and even peaceful, but mine had only caused panic and sadness. In the book "Grief Dreams," Wray writes that "grief dreams allow us to reconnect with our deceased loved ones, to return to that place where nothing has changed—a place where our loved one is still alive—a place where grief does not exist."[21] According to Wray, there are four types of grief dreams:

- **The visitation dream** - This type of dream involves the dreamer spending time with the deceased. They appear to the bereaved person in the dream, often without saying anything.

- **The message dream** - The dreamer receives information, instruction, or warning from the loved one. These messages may be about their own death or the death of the dreamer. They may also warn of an impending event that will occur.

- **The reassurance dream** - This dream can reassure the dreamer the deceased has made the transition and is happy or that they are proud of the dreamer. These are usually pleasant dreams and allow the person who is grieving to wake up feeling at peace.

- **The trauma dream** – This type of dream, while less common than the others, often includes flashbacks and is more likely to occur in the early stages of grief and when the death is traumatic.[22]

Despite my hope that my dreams about Dad would stop, I had another one in the second year after his death. I dreamed I was talking to someone, and I turned around and Dad was standing there. He had a small amount of blood on his face. He was dressed in a suit, and he looked like he was going to church. I leaned in to hug him, and his coat felt cold to my face. I laid my head on his chest, and he vanished. When I woke up, my face was cold from the ceiling fan. It was not traumatic like the other two dreams, but not really reassuring either. He was just gone. Just like in real life.

Interestingly, Wray reports most people come to eventually view their trauma dreams as helpful because they help them accept the reality of the loss, work through the various feelings and emotions, and help with the painful adjustment of living without the person they loved. While trauma dreamers are initially distressed, eventually, they view their trauma dreams as positive.[23] I'm not sure I'm there yet.

Sometimes, dreams take place during the day in the form of auditory or visual hallucinations of the deceased person, especially during the acute stage of grief.[24] It is not uncommon for the grieving person to hear familiar sounds that pertain to the loved one who has passed away or to get lost in thought about them coming back again. Henry Wadsworth Longfellow wrote a poem originally titled "Evening Shadows." There is a reference in the fourth stanza to his friend and brother-in-law, George W. Pierce. Of George he said, "I have never ceased to feel that in his death something was taken from my own life which could never be restored." The news of his friend and brother-in-law's death reached Mr. Longfellow in Heidelberg on Christmas Eve, 1835, less than a month after the death of Mrs. Longfellow who died during a miscarriage. The poem was later renamed "Footsteps of Angels."

This is a portion of that poem:

> *With a slow and noiseless footstep*
> *Comes that messenger divine,*
> *Takes the vacant chair beside me,*
> *Lays her gentle hand in mine.*

> *And she sits and gazes at me*
> *With those deep and tender eyes,*
> *Like the stars, so still and saint-like,*
> *Looking downward from the skies.*

Uttered not, yet comprehended,
Is the spirit's voiceless prayer,
Soft rebukes, in blessings ended,
Breathing from her lips of air. [25]

CHAPTER EIGHT

WHEN CHILDREN GRIEVE

As hard as my dad's death was, telling the children and grandchildren in our family added a new layer of pain to an already unbearable situation. The newest generations of our large family included young adults and teenagers, several elementary-school-aged kids, preschoolers, and a baby. It's hard to be therapeutic with children when you are consumed by grief yourself, but they needed to be told—and we needed to be the ones telling them. Because Dad was so involved with his grandchildren and his great-grandchildren, we knew the loss would be enormous. Often, children who are the same age may be in very different places developmentally, so our approach had to vary with each child. Helping them integrate the loss into their worldview was critical.

Most children are aware of death, even if they don't understand it. Two-thirds of children will experience the death of someone close to them by the age of ten, and 5% will experience the death of a parent by the age of sixteen. Their reactions to death are as varied as they are. Some may withdraw from regular activities, and very young children may revert to earlier activities such as thumb-sucking or bedwetting. Many researchers document the importance of positive caregiver relationships for decreasing mental health issues such as anxiety and depression. A safe physical environment where the child feels supported is critical.[26] It is interesting to note that the post-death environment is an important predictor of a child's mental health.[27]

When younger children grieve, they approach it very differently than adults. Specifically, they tend to demonstrate less withdrawal, depression, anxiety, or attention-related struggles than older kids. This age group also tends to demonstrate emotionality for shorter periods of time.[28] They may play and then cry for a short period of time before returning to play again. These "bursts" are common in the grieving child.

Sometimes children don't have the prerequisites to process grief. They may lack the knowledge and experience needed to fully comprehend what is taking place. That doesn't mean they don't experience sadness. Even babies have been shown to have symptomology consistent with mourning. They may lose weight, be clingy, have trouble sleeping, or be irritable. However, prior to the age of three, they usually do not have an understanding of death. Generally, between the ages of five and nine, children begin to comprehend the finality of death. After age ten, most children can understand that death is final, inevitable, and associated with the cessation of bodily activities.[29]

In all age groups, children may need the parent or family member to be nearby, reassure them through touch and comfort, or be available for discussion of the events that led to the death. Those discussions will change based on the age of the child. They often have many questions, as ours did. One thing we noticed was that different age groups had trouble at different times. The seven- and eight-year-olds had trouble at the time of his death, while the five- and six-year-olds had trouble a year later. This probably had to do with maturation and the ability to process and understand information.

Some of the older kids worried that someone else in our family would die, something that had never really crossed their minds before. This common response is an example of availability heuristics. The heuristic assumes that people infer the distal criterion (i.e., event frequency) by exploiting a proximal cue—namely, the mental availability of relevant instances.[30] To illustrate this concept, if you ask a group of people if they are more likely to die in a car accident or from a heart attack, they are more likely to name the event for which they have the most recent experience. They do this by recalling actual deaths within their proximate family or social network. It also leads them to overestimate the chances of the event happening again.

Affect heuristics works in much the same way, but emotion plays the lead role. Images of risk often come with strong emotional reactions that guide and inform risk judgments. In our case, fear amplified our kids' estimation of the risk that someone else would die. These two things caused them to disregard the truth (found in data) and come to their own conclusion. It's why even we as adults get risk wrong. These mental shortcuts allow us to decide quickly, but not always correctly. In any event, children may be reassured by a conversation about why they feel this way and why their fears are not facts. I am no more likely to die today than I was yesterday just because my dad died. Sometimes, that's a hard concept to get our heads around when the situation is so emotionally charged and the loss is so great.

For most of our children, my dad's passing was their first experience with the death of someone they loved. The realization of this loss came on gradually for some and immediately for others. The intensity of their grief was at times hard to decipher. Knowing how to best support them in the post-death environment was guesswork at best on most days. For a few of the children, grief counseling was beneficial. Even though it often felt—as parents and grandparents, aunts and uncles—we were stumbling down a dark and unknown path, we did the best we could to guide the children, even as we found a way for ourselves. Sometimes, all we could do was hold the light.

CHAPTER NINE

MOURNING IN THE DIGITAL AGE

We posted a notice of my dad's death on social media the day after he died. We didn't post anything from the time he collapsed until the morning following his death. I put a picture of him with the announcement. Oddly enough, it was a picture I took of him just six weeks prior for this exact purpose. It was of him right after he told me a joke and we were both laughing. He was so delighted with himself and my response to his joke, and I thought at the time, this is such a good representation of him." He was always saying something funny or laughing about something. He found humor in just about everything. It was a gift he gave me, and even right after he died, I thought of something funny.

We were leaving the hospital and my niece said, "We gave it the old college try."

The first thing that popped into my head was, "Yeah, and just like OSU (his beloved Oklahoma State Cowboys), he couldn't get it to the goal line."

My niece just looked at me and said, "Grandpa would have laughed at that." I knew he would have been proud of me for going to humor first.

I chose the words for the announcement carefully. This would be the first time most of our friends and extended family would hear the news, and I wanted it to be gentle and meaningful. The outpouring of sympathy and love was immediate. It was easier than contacting people individually and—quite frankly—none of us were in any shape to retell the story over and over. It was a blessing to be able to communicate our loss in this distant, detached manner. The condolences were heartfelt and comforting. This public dissemination of news is one benefit of social networking sites.

Prior to my dad's death, digital mourning was something to which I had never given much thought. In the weeks and months following his death, I began researching this new way to grieve, finding a moderate body of literature on the subject. Mourning a loved one has always been considered one of the most painful human experiences we will face, but the way we mourn is changing. I discovered mourning is undergoing a metamorphosis, and as a society we are gradually adapting to these changes. Our relationship with grief is much like that of past generations, but the way we express that grief is different.

In the article "Mourning with Social Media: Rewiring Grief," the authors say a coping mechanism unique to the twenty-first century is grieving through social media.[31] In the days that followed my dad's death, social media was oddly comforting to me. We were able to post his passing and let others know about the details of the service. Many people took the time to offer condolences, as well as share stories about him that meant so much to us. In this way, social media can make us feel less isolated and more connected to those who knew our loved one.

When someone we love dies, it's hard to understand how the world continues to turn, why we seem to be the only one suffering. Grief is a very isolating experience. Our pain is so acute, so vivid, it is difficult to comprehend how others go about their business while we are paralyzed. In conversations with people who are or who have been in mourning, they all say the same thing. They were shocked that people around them continued on with their lives, going to work, shopping, doing normal things. How could such trauma exist when so many others were simply unaffected? It reminds me of the F5 tornados that struck the nearby community of Moore, Oklahoma, on two occasions. There were neighborhoods where one house was completely gone, yet another house just next door was untouched. I thought about that a lot in the days after my dad's death. The death of a loved one can feel like a direct hit from a tornado. That's why social media can be therapeutic. There is often comfort in the fact that somebody else in the world understands our pain.[32] It helps to know that someone knew our loved one and felt that loss as well. It is somehow validating that the person we loved mattered, that their life counted for something, that they might be remembered by someone other than ourselves.

Digital mourning is a new concept, and has yet to be fully explored, but one study found "people mourn online not necessarily to remember the dead, but to personally grieve."[33] This "do-it-yourself" mourning is gaining in popularity. Many young, middle-aged, and older adults now use social media platforms daily. They use this medium as a resource for many different areas in their lives. Mourning online is a natural progression for these individuals.

For many people, grief is an experience processed without professional help. Social media can be the therapy they turn to. This is especially true of grief in the younger generation, where technology and its use are an integral part of their everyday lives. For many, an experience with death at this age may be their first exposure to mortality. Turning to technology can be a natural outlet for their grief.[34]

Digital platforms are a way for people from all walks of life to come together and share their similar interests.[35] Having a place to express grief and to receive condolences from others can aid in healing and can also serve as a written memorial. Writing allows the individual to experience peace through the processing of emotion while also creating a public record that others may find useful in their own grief journey. Online mourning can support our grief when we are feeling disenfranchised by the process. The words we write or the words we read can resonate through a commonality that might not be available elsewhere. The advent of social media platforms like Facebook, Instagram, and other networking sites allows for this expression of grief.[36] Something as complicated as the grief experience often requires a wide range of resources to adequately address the loss. Heraclitus's famous quote—"No man ever steps in the same river twice, for it's not the same river and he's not the same man"—applies to grief. Every death is different, every person is different, and the same person may experience the death of someone they love differently with each new encounter of loss. Social media can be a valid part of that process.

After the death of her husband David, Facebook's COO, Sheryl Sandberg, moved to create a *legacy contact,* which enables a user, pre-death, to name someone to run their profile. The appointed individual would have the ability to memorialize the page. They can also take the page down if the deceased person instructed prior to death they did not want to maintain a digital presence.

As of 2016, there were well over 30 million profiles for deceased users still on Facebook's site with as many as eight thousand more users dying daily.[37] Of the deceased profiles still running, many continue to have new comments, likes, or visits. This further supports research that found value in maintaining these sites. This grief communication helps mourners navigate their own grief journey. It may also be a way to financially support the survivors through links to organizations like GoFundMe. Social networking sites can be a virtual crowdsourcing for grief.

Technology can also normalize grief. It can make grief more visible, resulting in comfort and support for the bereaved. This dialog with the dead, although one-sided, can be therapeutic. It can help us renegotiate our bond with the deceased, post-death. More recent grief models support the idea of continuing bonds with the dead as opposed to older, more traditional models that advocated recovery was best achieved by a relative disconnection from the loved one. This approach can help us readjust to the new environment while forging a new, different connection to the dead.[38]

Past research has shown that funerals help the bereaved in the short term, but there is little known benefit to this ritual in the long term. This is where online grieving can be beneficial.[39] When the rest of the world has moved on, the grieving person can come back, much like visiting a grave, only the flowers they leave take the form of words. After the loss of her son, my friend Amy said, "When they are born, we measure their days in minutes and hours first, then days and weeks, then months. We measure their death in the same way." Social media is a way to say, "I know it's been six months, but I still grieve, he still mattered, and I still need support." Virtual grieving can give visibility to the pain we feel privately. With more than one billion users worldwide, Facebook and other platforms like it will be a vital part of the grieving process for many. For some, this way of communication can make the loss more bearable.

CHAPTER TEN

WHEN GRIEF RUNS DEEP

On a fall morning in 2015, NFL legend Doug Flutie's dad passed way. One hour later, his mother collapsed and died. Doug Flutie said he believed his mother died of a broken heart.[40] There have been many stories just like this, but is it more than just coincidence that two people who have been together for so long die in such close proximity? During the grief process after my dad died, I began to think about the physiological response of the mourner's body to loss. Could there be a neurobiological reason why we become more susceptible to illness and death in the days and months following the loss of a loved one? Even though children and young adults often overestimate the probability of death based on availability heuristics, it has long been anecdotally held that grief can contribute to the illness or death of an older surviving spouse. Recent research suggests there may be science behind this phenomenon.

One condition that can result from grief is takotsubo cardiomyopathy, more commonly known as broken-heart syndrome. This condition is a weakening of the left ventricle, which is the heart's main pumping chamber. This is generally brought on as the result of severe emotional or physical stress, such as a sudden illness, the loss of a loved one, a serious accident, or other severe stressors. Scientists surmise it is caused by a sudden surge of hormones that basically "stun" the heart. Older women may be particularly susceptible to this phenomenon because of reduced levels of estrogen after menopause. Research on rats that had their ovaries removed, but that were given estrogen during periods of stress, fared better than those without the protective hormone. They also had less left-ventricle dysfunction and higher levels of certain heart-protective substances.[41] It is widely accepted that the death of a spouse is one of the most stressful life events a person will experience. In medicine, it is well-documented that stress hormones such as cortisol, epinephrine, and norepinephrine that are raised by grief or other stressors can take a damaging toll on the body.

Researchers at the University of Birmingham in the United Kingdom found age alters the body's immune system so that younger people are more resilient when it comes to the grief experience, while older people become more susceptible to infection. In this study, the researchers looked at the effect of bereavement on neutrophil function. Neutrophils are the white blood cells essential to fighting infection in the body. They also examined the stress hormones cortisol and dehydroepiandrosterone sulfate (DHEAS). Elderly people in the study showed reduced immune function, higher stress hormone levels, and weaker neutrophil function compared to their younger counterparts. Around the age of thirty, the amount of DHEAS naturally begins to decline, eventually resulting in elderly patients possessing only 20% of the normal levels of this hormone by the time they reach old age. This is a significant finding because DHEAS balances out cortisol. Without this check and balance system, cortisol levels climb in the body, allowing inflammation to gain the upper hand.[42] The researchers suggested the possibility of a DHEAS supplement for those who are grieving. Further studies need to be conducted to ascertain if the addition of this supplement will provide needed protection during the vulnerable time period when patient risk for morbidity and mortality is at its highest.

In a nine-year study, researchers collected data from 373,189 elderly married couples, looking specifically at morbidity and mortality after one of the spouses died. For men whose wives died first, there was an 18% increase in all-cause mortality, and there was a 16% increase for women. One longitudinal study put the highest risk for death at more than 30% in the first three months. Those statistics fell to 15% in the months that followed the acute phase of grief.[43] Other studies have replicated this data. A study of 4,000 couples at the University of Glasgow found that, on average, both older men and women were at least 30% more likely to die of any cause in the first six months following a spouse's death than those who hadn't lost a partner. An additional large study in Jerusalem placed this risk closer to 50%. Dr. Lee Lipsenthal said sudden death from pre-existing heart disease is the number one cause of death in a grieving spouse, with the risk extending through the first eighteen months after the death of the spouse.[44]

This widowhood effect, as it is referred to, is widely accepted by the medical community. The relationship between stress and inflammation is well understood and is thought to be contributory to this increase in grief-associated morbidity. While the acute phase of grief is the most dangerous for complications and poor outcomes, some studies show a nine-year timeline to be realistic for complete recovery. In some patients, who may be more genetically predisposed and more vulnerable to circulating elevated inflammatory markers, the risk for death may be more likely.[45]

In addition to an increased risk of morbidity and mortality following the death of a loved one, there is also a list of symptoms that accompany the grieving process. While these symptoms are not as serious as those in the previously noted research, they are still bothersome to the person who experiences them. In his book "A Grief Observed," C.S. Lewis describes symptoms such as fluttering in his stomach, restlessness, yawning, and too much swallowing.[46]

In the weeks after my dad's death, I found myself sighing. A lot. My mother mentioned the same symptom in herself. This was also observed by Erich Lindemann, who was the chief of psychiatry at Massachusetts General Hospital at the time of his research in the 1940s. Prior to his 1944 groundbreaking study on the 1942 Cocoanut Grove fire, he studied patients who had lost body parts from disease or trauma. Interestingly, he referred to this as "partial death." This, he told the medical residents, forces the patient to figure out a new life without the missing thing. He surmised the loss precipitated grief and that the patient needed to find a way to function without the missing part. It required the person to rethink how they could relate to a constellation of altered social ties. This was the perfect prelude to his research with family members of the victims after the Cocoanut Grove fire. This tragedy remains America's deadliest nightclub fire, and, until 9/11, it was the second-deadliest single-building fire in United

States history.[47] His work with these families would change the way we collectively think about grief. The term "partial death" exactly describes what I felt happen to me when my dad died.

Dr. Lindemann's 1944 research explored symptomology in family members of those killed in the fire. He reported "sensations of somatic distress occurring in waves lasting from twenty minutes to an hour at a time, a feeling of tightness in the throat, choking with shortness of breath, need for sighing, and an empty feeling in the abdomen, lack of muscular power, and an intense subjective distress described as tension or mental pain."[48] His reference to the "need for sighing" and my own experience with the same got me thinking about the physiological basis for this respiratory anomaly.

Lindemann said one of the most striking features of grief is the marked tendency to sighing respirations.[49] According to a study done at the University of Leuven, sighs are the body's way of reacting to a negative mood. They can also be associated with boredom, disappointment, defeat, and longing. The hypothesis is that sighing is a psychophysiological reset. It could also advance coping with high-arousal and/or negative emotional states. Sighs have been specifically related to changes in respiratory variability. They also restore a balance between random respiratory variability and respirations that are correlated to physical or emotional states. Since increased total respiratory variability and reduced correlated respiratory variability are characteristic of negative and/ or high-arousal emotional states, this could explain the increased sigh rates during these emotions. Finally, restoration of a balance between random and correlated respiratory variability co-occurs with a feeling of relief. Accordingly, sighs may improve coping with negative and high-arousal states, and may relieve tension, restlessness, and stress. Sighing may simply be the body's way of attempting a reset.[50]

In addition to the respiratory system, the prolonged activation of other bodily systems can result in a variety of symptoms experienced by the person who is grieving. This can take the form of generalized fatigue, muscle tension and aches, gastric symptoms, migraines, and sometimes mental disorders.[51] In my work with sexual-assault patients, I have noted a commonality of abdominal pain in this population in the immediate aftermath of the assault. Without an external, identifiable injury to attribute this discomfort to, I have come to believe it is likely ascribed to the increase in stress hormones and their effect on the abdominal muscles. This muscle tension is common in both trauma and grief. In his research, Eric Lindemann eventually concludes that grief is brutally physiological. I came to that conclusion as well.

On a February morning in 1972, Dr. Lindemann addressed a group of doctors and nurses—this time, not as their teacher, but rather their patient. These physicians had spent the previous six years treating him for a sacral chordoma, a rare cancer occurring in the lower back. With little time left, he faced his own personal loss. He wanted them to understand that all the research he had done throughout his career helped him see more clearly a pathway through grief, even if that grief was his own. He was facing death as an expert on the subject. He said the thing that hits you is that you realize you are not immortal.

Another problem, in his opinion, that caused further trauma for the patients and their families was that the staff felt limited in their time and emotional resources. It was easier to view the patient as a biological specimen. This depersonalization is exactly what we experienced with the physician who seemed too busy to be bothered with us when Dad was dying. Dr. Lindemann told those present that day that patients had the need to be heard—they need to talk. They often need to reconstruct their identity, to paint a picture of who they were. Families need time to work through the process as well. In those hard, traumatic moments, what patients and their families need most is our time as healthcare professionals. This is the kind of care they need. Lindemann told his doctors, "One can be surprised at how little actual time expenditure is needed to say the right word at the right time, and not too much."[52] As Dr. Lindemann was dying, he knew what he needed from his healthcare team. I wish my dad's doctor had known—we needed that, too.

CHAPTER ELEVEN

KICKING AGAINST THE BOTTOM

Once, when I was young, maybe seven or eight, my family went on vacation. The morning we were leaving to return home, we begged Mom and Dad to let us swim just once more before we loaded the car and got back on the road. After some time, we must have worn them down, because they relented. We put our bathing suits on, still damp from the night before, and we went for one final swim. The water was clear blue and sparkled in the morning sun.

I couldn't wait. The first thing I did was climb to the top of the slide. Before my dad even knew what was happening, I was coming down hard and fast, gaining momentum as I quickly made my way toward the center of the pool. Just before I slipped under the water, I heard him yell, "That's the deep end!" Down I went, sinking like a rock. There was sudden silence as the water filled my ears and eyes. My delight turned to sheer panic when I realized I couldn't swim. The weight of the water seemed to push me further and further down until my feet finally hit the bottom of the pool. There was a fleeting moment when I thought there would be no escape and I would die at the bottom of that pool. On vacation. In my favorite bathing suit.

I used every bit of strength I had left to push off the bottom. Just when I didn't think I could hold my breath any longer, my head broke the surface of the pool and I gasped for air, before quickly sinking again. I flailed about in the water, alternating between the surface and just below it. I thought I was drowning. I probably was. My dad stood at the edge of the pool, already dressed for the trip home. He was not happy. There was a teenage boy close by, and my dad calmly said, "Can you grab her for me?" He grabbed me from behind and towed me to the side, where Dad quickly reached down with one hand and pulled me out. I didn't care how much trouble I was in; I was just so thankful he had pulled me to safety.

As I progressed through the grieving process, I thought about this experience and how grief was like being at the bottom of that pool when I was young. It can feel like you are suffocating, like the weight of the water just keeps pushing you further and further down. You just keep sinking, and you feel like there may not even be a bottom to find.

Research tell us that 75% of the population will experience a traumatic event at some point in their lives.[53] For many of us, this trauma will be the death of a loved one. The way we eventually deal with this experience will determine how well we adjust in the aftermath. There is evidence to suggest the effects of trauma might not be exclusively negative. Trauma brings about change, of this we are certain, but a wide body of research reveals change can encompass a positive outcome if we can kick against the bottom and rise to the top.

The field of positive psychology, posttraumatic growth (PTG) has been the focus of trauma recovery for some time. PTG is a positive change experienced as a result of the struggle with a major life crisis or a traumatic event. In fact, as many as 90% of survivors report at least one aspect of PTG, such as a renewed appreciation for life. While not the first to discuss PTG, Richard Tedeschi and Lawrence Calhoun[54] have done much to systematize investigation into the topic. They have identified five major domains of PTG:

- **Appreciation of life** – People often set new priorities. They have a greater appreciation for the smaller things in life and may redefine how they want to spend their days and with whom.

- **Relating to others** - Warmer, more intimate relationships often form after trauma. They may feel a closer connection to family or friends.

- **Personal strength** - The person has a cognitive reconstruction because of the trauma. They feel better able to handle adversity and have a new sense of awareness of self, are more empathetic, creative, mature, and may even be humbler. They are also more vulnerable, having experienced trauma, possibly understanding for the first time that they have no real control over some events.

- **New possibilities** – This can include a changed philosophy and meaning-making out of trauma. Often the individual begins to look at ways to make contributions to society and may change what things are meaningful or important to them.

- **Spiritual change** – Many people report a deeper relationship with God, but even if they don't believe, they may still report some spiritual growth.

PTG can be a good, albeit unintended, result of trauma and loss. The Cocoanut Grove fire is an example of this. Physicians, forced to be innovative, discovered new burn treatments for their patients. Those treatments are still used today. Building design and safety codes were changed because of the 492 lives lost and the 150 injured that night. Pioneering psychologist Alexandra Adler was among the first to write detailed papers on post-traumatic stress syndrome, using information drawn from her studies of the surviving victims of the fire. Many of the survivors were left with permanent brain damage, which prompted her to study anxiety and depression after catastrophes, later applying her findings to the treatment of World War II veterans. And of course, Erich Lindemann's first-ever systematic study of grief led to the understanding of survivor grief.[55] These were all positive outgrowths of tragedy.

The Saturday after my dad's death, we met at my parents' house. Really, at that point, it was just my mom's house. I had been thinking about an idea to honor my dad's life since the night we spent in the hospital. Because there were so many nurses in our family and because my parents were always helping someone, I thought we should create a nursing scholarship to honor them and to help nursing students. A few weeks before my dad died, a lifelong friend of our family had passed away. When his daughters found out we had created the scholarship, they wanted to donate a portion of their parent's estate to the cause. The Jim & Judy Archer and Ed & Eva Pope Endowed Nursing Scholarship was created. This has been our PTG. Helping to establish this scholarship and meeting the recipients has been an important part of the healing process for Mom, myself, my sisters, and the Pope sisters. We couldn't think of a better way to continue our parents' spirit of giving and service to others. This scholarship stands as a testament to the potential growth that can be experienced after loss. Resilience is important when we experience trauma, but it only gets us back to where we were before the traumatic event. PTG propels us forward. It goes beyond resilience and helps us recover, and if we are diligent in our effort, we can be better versions of our old selves.

Dr. Viktor Frankl found this to be true as well. He was an Austrian neurologist and psychiatrist as well as a Holocaust survivor. He authored the bestselling *Man's Search for Meaning* based on his experiences in the death camps. During his time of captivity, he discovered the importance of finding meaning in all forms of existence, even the most brutal ones. He said forces beyond your control can take away everything you possess except one thing: your freedom to choose how you will respond to the situation. He also felt any man who has a *Why* to live can bear almost any *How*.[56] He carefully chose his response to the hard circumstances he faced in Auschwitz and found it was the only thing he really could control. Finding meaning, even in the worst situations, can bring peace. Dr. Frankl found it, and it became my quest as well.

CHAPTER TWELVE

FINDING GRATITUDE IN GRIEF

In the months following my dad's death, it was hard to sort through my emotions. The sadness, anxiety, and anger were prevalent, but slowly, a new emotion began to make its way into my subconscious. I remember being in church one Sunday morning and feeling overwhelmed with gratefulness for Dad. Thankful he had taken us to church, thankful for my faith, appreciative for the care and sacrifice he had given our family. I wondered how gratitude might change the discussion around grief.

Several research studies have identified that feelings of gratitude are correlated with lower heart rate, lower blood pressure, and improved immune functioning. Other studies have established that gratitude toward God results in a better capacity to cope more effectively with the deleterious effects of stress.[57] The word gratitude is derived from the Latin root gratia, meaning grace, graciousness, or gratefulness. All derivatives of this Latin word have to do with kindness, generousness, gifts, giving, receiving, or getting something for nothing.[58] Zig Ziglar said, "Gratitude is the healthiest of all emotions." [59] Gratitude is, quite simply put, a state of thankfulness.

What does science have to say about gratitude and its transforming power on the body and mind? We know there are neural mechanisms responsible for feelings of gratitude. Studies have identified the right anterior temporal cortex of the brain as the birthplace for moral judgments involving feelings of gratefulness.[60] The use of gratitude acts as a natural antidepressant. When we express gratitude, our brain releases dopamine and serotonin, the two crucial neurotransmitters responsible for our emotions. These chemicals make us feel good.

The same research found differences in the central nervous system of people who express and feel gratitude compared to those who don't. Those who were more grateful in their daily lives had a higher volume of grey matter in parts of the brain. Grey matter is home to our emotions; it serves to process information in the brain. The grey matter includes regions of the brain involved in muscle control and sensory perception such as seeing and hearing, memory, emotions, speech, decision making, and self-control. But even if we don't biologically have an increased amount of grey matter, we can cultivate it by consciously practicing gratitude every day. We can help these neural pathways to strengthen themselves and ultimately create a permanent grateful and positive nature within ourselves.[61] Further research suggests that meditation can have a powerful effect on the brain's structure. The authors point to the brain's remarkable plasticity and how environmental enrichment has been shown to remodel the brain.[62] Prayer can have the same effect in that it is also a mindful activity. This re-mapping of the brain can be a result of focused and mindful gratitude.

Gratitude has also been defined as "the willingness to recognize the unearned increments of value in one's experience."[63] Unearned increments of value—I thought a lot about that statement. Twenty-eight years prior to my dad's death, when I was still the young mother of a three-year-old child, I had gone to the doctor because I was coughing up blood. After much testing and many delays, I was diagnosed with a carcinoid tumor. I would need to have surgery to prevent spread of the disease. After that hard discussion with my physician, I left his office, went to the parking lot, and sat in my car. So much anxiety, so much fear. I was only twenty-five years old. I put my key in the ignition and turned the car on. The clock flashed 11:17. I had the distinct impression the message to me was I needed to live at 11:17, not 11:18. I needed to stop worrying about what was going to happen the next minute, the next day, the next year. The physical address of my house at the time was 1117. I felt strongly impressed by the thought that I didn't need to worry about what was going on in the house next door. They lived at 1119. What happened at that house next door was out of my control, even though it might have a profound effect on my life. Through the years, through the reoccurrence of my tumor and the subsequent loss of my lung, I would come to see that number as a gentle reminder that I am not in control, that I must trust that "all things work together for good to those who love God" (Rom 8:28).

Twenty-eight years later, my dad would collapse on 11/16/17. I didn't even realize what the date was at the time, but on the morning of the day he died, when I went home to change clothes, I flipped my phone over to check the time—11:17 on 11/17/17. In that instant, I knew that this would be the day he would die. Could it be knowing how I would struggle with guilt over Dad's death, that I had given a gift years earlier, so I would know that his day of death was already appointed? That there was nothing I could do to move that event to the right or left. My gratitude for that *unearned increment of value* was very real in that moment. Even though I would question his death over the next two years,

1117 became a touchstone in my life. A place to return to until I could internalize its message.

I began to think about the other things I was grateful for, such as the fact that the night he collapsed outside, on the driveway, it was unseasonably warm. In November, it should have been cold. The extended family was in town for a family picture, but the picture was never the reason we were all there. We were allowed this mercy of being present as a family, all thirty of us, to say goodbye. I have so much gratitude for that, even if we didn't get one last photo. I am thankful that of all the firemen who could have responded to that 911 call, it was someone we knew, someone Dad knew. Someone who cared about us. I am thankful I felt him slipping away that summer, and I was allowed extra time to say goodbye even though his death, when it came, was sudden. I am thankful for the gift of 1117, twenty-eight years in advance.

I found the more I sought out gratitude, the more I genuinely *felt* grateful. Research studies confirm that gratitude is effective in increasing well-being because it builds psychological, social, and spiritual resources, and inspires prosocial reciprocity.[64] Finding things to be thankful for was healing, and in a way that was easier than I would have thought. The more I sought gratitude, the more it found me.

CHAPTER THIRTEEN

TO COMFORT ALWAYS

E dward Livingston Trudeau was an American physician who established the Adirondack Cottage Sanitarium for the treatment of tuberculosis in the 1800s. He became interested in the treatment of the disease as a teenager. During that time, he cared for his older brother, who would eventually succumb to the illness after a three-year battle. One of Dr. Trudeau's four children died of pneumonia, two others from tuberculosis. He himself would ultimately die from the same disease. He knew great heartache and struggle, as a lot of those from his generation did.

In an op-ed piece written in the New York Times shortly after his death in 1915, a former patient wrote of Dr. Trudeau, "he always lightened the load, even when he could not lift it." He was known as the Beloved Physician.[65] The saying, "To cure sometimes, to relieve often, and to comfort always," ascribed to Dr. Trudeau and others, encapsulates his sympathetic engagement with patient suffering.

Dr. Abraham Verghese is an American physician and professor who, through his extensive practice and writing, became influential in the art of medicine as a ministry of healing. Early in his career, he noted the importance of communication, touch, body language, and tone as fundamental components to the healing process. The patient-physician relationship, he proposed, was as important as the treatment prescribed. He encourages physicians to empathize with their patients and to see them individually. He advocates for healthcare workers to see patients and their families as human beings who are suffering, fearful, and in need not just of treatment, but of comfort and reassurance.[66]

A couple of weeks after my dad's death, my father-in-law was brought to the hospital by ambulance late in the evening. He was septic and in critical condition. I texted Wendy, who works in my pulmonologist's office, to see if she would ask Dr. Cook to stop by and check on my father-in-law the next morning. About thirty minutes later, he walked into the room where we were waiting for an ICU bed.

"What are you doing here this late?" I asked.

He quickly moved to the bedside and began assessing the situation in his calm, reassuring manner, something he has done thousands of times. With his back to me, he pulled his stethoscope out of his jacket and said, "I just didn't think this family needed any more stress, so I decided to come in tonight and take care of him myself." He bent over the bed and listened to my father-in-law's labored breathing.

When he was finished, he turned around and looked at me. He was tired; I could see it in his face. His day started before dawn that morning, as it usually does, seeing patients in the ICU, then a full patient load in his office. Winter is brutal for patients and the physicians who care for them. Still, he came. Nothing he could do that night would bring my dad back, but he chose to lighten our load even if he could not lift it.

There will not always be effective treatment or a cure for those who are dying, but there should always be comfort. Patients need that, families need that, we needed that. Dr. Lindemann, Dr. Trudeau, and Dr. Verghese knew that, even if my dad's physician didn't. His words, his indifference, his body language all said, "It's not going to matter," and for my dad's prognosis, he was correct. But in that moment, we all—my sisters, my mother, and me—became patients. We were suddenly in desperate need of a physician who, like Trudeau, could have chosen to "lighten our load, even if he could not lift it." Helping families in crisis is ultimately preventive medicine.

Some struggles I encountered in the aftermath of Dad's death were, I now know, predictable. Looking at the research helped me understand how trauma and grief affects the mind and body on a cellular level and, in some cases, can even lead to the death of the person who is grieving. It helped to know how grief permeates every aspect of our being. It seeps into the basement of our memories, each long-forgotten and seemingly unimportant event from our childhood adding another drop until we feel we might drown. I know now that falling down the rabbit hole of grief is common, expected, and *temporary*. Eventually, you do stop falling. While the pain in some form will always exist, the hole is not as dark and deep as it was in the beginning.

I better understand how grief compels us to retrace the events of the death, looking for details that might change the outcome. This magical thinking, I now know, happens often. The search for answers continues until our minds, overwhelmed and weary, begin the process of accepting what will not change. I know that guilt takes the lead in the early stages of grief and is far more common than I would have guessed. I also know we are not spared sadness, even in our dreams. But these visions, though often frightening, can help us process loss. Even when we are not consciously aware, our mind and body seek to stabilize and heal.

Eventually, grief becomes softer. These days, when I pass the hospital room where families go to hear bad news, I still wince in pain, but grief no longer screams at me from a white, plastic patient's belongings bag. It's more of a gentle nudge. When I look at the fence, broken on the night Dad collapsed, the new board is now almost indistinguishable from the older wood on either side, and I understand some scars we carry internally, even if no one else knows they are there.

Just as Dr. Frankl found meaning in a dirty, hope-deprived concentration camp, I have tried to find meaning in my dad's death. Dr. Frankl said, "If there is a meaning in life at all, then there must be a meaning in suffering. Suffering is an ineradicable part of life, even as fate and death."[67] After Dad's death, my family has tried to pursue PTG through the formation of a nursing scholarship and to create a lasting legacy by encouraging healthcare workers to care for families in crisis. We do this by training new nurses not simply in the technology of care, but in the best practice of caring. We want these families to have what we didn't receive. Finally, I have learned that gratitude is a gentler emotion and can soften the harshness of anger, anxiety, regret, and grief. It can also rewire our brains, so we can better cope during the painful period of readjustment. This point remains: our attitude is really the only thing we can control.

Recently, I was taking care of a patient in the emergency department when an older, grey-haired man was rolled in on a stretcher. He had been at home when he collapsed. He was in cardiac arrest. I knew his chances of surviving, like my dad's, were six percent. His family waited in a room nearby. Even though I couldn't see them, I internalized their anxiety. I listened as the medical team tried to save his life, ultimately and predictably calling the time of death. I don't know if his family was being updated during the resuscitation or how they were informed of his death, but I hope it was with care, compassion, and comfort. I hope a nurse and physician went in the room, sat down, talked, and listened. I hope they touched them, that there was some kind of physical contact. I hope instead of hands on their hips and their body turned away, they faced that family and gave them the gift of time and attention. Ultimately, in that moment of crisis, all we as healthcare professionals have left to offer is comfort. Our duty to that patient who has died is over, but our obligation to lighten the load, even if we cannot lift it, has just begun. Every family that is forced to say goodbye to their loved one and leave the hospital with a white, plastic bag deserves our comfort. Always.

HEALING

It's been almost two years. Two Christmases have passed. We struggled through them both. Two springs came and went, and two summers turned to fall. Three kids went off to college and another began to walk, teetering at first, but quickly gaining balance. Extraordinary and ordinary days slipped by as we moved slowly forward. When the loss was fresh, I wished for the days to speed by, to quickly move me away from those painful events. I thought time and distance were the answer, but in some ways, they made grief more complicated. What I didn't count on— what I failed to understand—was with every passing day, he was getting farther and farther away, like a ship moving toward the horizon. When I accidently erased his voice mail, I cried. I was forgetting what he sounded like. In the growing space between us, he was getting harder to find, beginning to disappear in the hazy distance where the sea meets the sky.

In the beginning, I hung on to Kübler Ross's five stages of grief. "This is a good idea," I thought. "I can move quickly through the stages and check them off my list." I love a good list and a yellow highlighter. I can't even have gum in my purse because I feel like I need to get it chewed and get it out of there. But with grief, things rarely move in a straight line. Grief has its own timeline and it's very rarely ours.

I found comfort in odd places. One day late in the fall, our water heater went out. I told my husband I wished my dad were here; he would know who to call. Because he was a builder, he usually handled these things. We went out to the garage to find out what type of heater we would need. When I opened the door to the closet, there inside, in his own handwriting, was the date it was installed: 11/17/11. Exactly six years before the day he died. It felt it was like a message that he was still there in tangible ways (although there was still no instruction on what kind of water heater to buy). I think these messages are always around us if we look, and grief makes us more available to them. Maybe our minds are less cluttered; maybe we see connections more clearly. Perhaps time and distance give us new perspectives.

This was certainly true for Elizabeth, the queen mother. After the death of her husband King George IV, she mourned his loss for six months, rarely being seen in public. After encouragement from Winston Churchill, she began to emerge from her mourning, and she said, "How small and selfish is sorrow and it bangs about until one is senseless." When someone asked her if grief gets better, she said, "It doesn't get better, but you get better at it."[68]

I got better at it, too. My experience with grief changed me in many ways. For one thing, grief made me more empathetic to those who are experiencing loss. As a clinician, I now understand what lies ahead for my patients' families. I know the trauma of death proceeds the hard days that follow. I underestimated those days and the effort it would take to move forward. I also came to understand there are choices, even in loss. There are ways out of the darkness even if those paths are hard to find. Ultimately, we choose how to move forward from the oppressive sadness. I think Queen Elizabeth was right; sorrow is small and selfish, and though it feels like a betrayal to the person who has died, finding ways to enjoy life again is the only healthy option. It will take a while, but eventually you will have more good days than bad. Mourning is simply an act of endurance, and I learned to trust the process of grief.

To the healthcare providers who give us the hardest news, it is important to understand-that you have the power to change the trajectory of healing. Do it carefully. Do it with compassion. Your job does not end with the death of the patient—in many ways, it is just beginning. Helping these families with end-of-life decisions brings clarity in the days to come when guilt will cloud their memories and make them second-guess their actions. Those internal discussions will come, and those who grieve will retrace every conversation, every action. You have the ability to give them the gift of peace, and no amount of money can buy that when sadness settles in and stays.

In this second year after the death of my dad, a hole remains. I suspect it always will. In the beginning, the pain seemed so localized, but we soon realized, that was a gross misunderstanding of the collateral nature of our loss. I underestimated the weight of grief and the strength needed to carry it. What I didn't anticipate was the role gratitude would play in my healing. He left too soon—I will always feel that way—but gratitude has a transforming power to gradually move us from a place where sadness is suffocating to a place of thankfulness. One researcher attributes gratefulness to the operation of a scarcity heuristic. This means we value things more when they are rare or scarce. So, when we face death or experience the death of a loved one, we realize that life is precious and the value we place on it rises.[69] My research (or as we call it, "me search") kept coming back to this phenomenon. Being thankful elevates us. It's a simple concept with powerful implications.

I will always be grateful for the time I had with him. I will always be sad he is gone. But just as he is woven into the very DNA of every cell in my body, even his death has made me better. I would expect nothing less from him.

ENDNOTES

1   Kubler-Ross, E., & Kessler, D. (2005). *On grief and grieving*. New York, NY: Scribner.

2   Didion, J. (2005). *The year of magical thinking*. New York, NY: Random House. P4

3   Leske, J. S., McAndrew, N. S., & Brasel, K. J. (2013, April-June). Experiences of families when present during resuscitation in the emergency department after trauma. *Journal of Trauma Nursing*, 20(2), 77-85.

4   Ravid, S., Shorer, S., Reshef, A., Schiff, E., Shacham, M., Cohen, L., & Bloch, B. (2019, February). Treatment of Post-Traumatic Stress Disorder using integrative medicine: Case history. *Journal of Chinese Medicine* , *119*, 5-12.

5   Graham, R., McCoy, M., & Schultz, A. (Eds.). (2015). *Strategies to improve cardiac arrest survival: A time to act*. Washington DC: The National Academies Press.

6   Alves, E., Lukoyanov, N., Serrao, P., Moura, D., & Moreira-Rodrigues, M. (2016). Epinephrine increases contextual learning through activation of peripheral β-adrenoceptors. *Psychopharmacology*, *233*(11), 2099–2108. https://doi.org/10.1007/s00213-016-4254-5

7   Sandberg, S., & Grant, A. (2017). *Option B: Facing adversity, building resilience, and finding joy*. New York: Alfred A. Knopf.

8   Kubler-Ross, E., & Kessler, D. (2005). *On grief and grieving*. New York, NY: Scribner. P. xxi

9   Enright, E. (1938). *Thimble Summer*. New York, NY: Henry Holt.

10 Kubler-Ross, E., & Kessler, D. (2005). *On grief and grieving*. New York, NY: Scribner.

11 Lewis, C. S. (1961). *A Grief Observed*. New York, NY: HarperCollins. P.3

12 Klass, D., & Steffen, E. M. (2018). *Continuing bonds In bereavement: New directions for research and practice*. New York, NY: Routledge, Taylor & Francis.

13 Walter, T. (1996). Bereavement and biography. *Mortality*, 1(1), 7-25.

14 Levy, A. (1999). *The orphaned adult: Understanding and coping with grief and change after the death of our parents*. Cambridge, MA: Da Capo Press. P.7

15 Levy, A. (1999). *The orphaned adult: Understanding and coping with grief and change after the death of our parents*. Cambridge, MA: Da Capo Press. P. 15

16 Shakespeare, W. (1997). *Hamlet* 1.2.290-295 Evans. G. Ed. Boston: Houghton Mifflin

17 Sharpless, B. A., & Grom, J. L. (2016). Isolated sleep paralysis: fear, prevention, and disruption. *Behavioral Sleep Medicine, 14,* (2) 134-139. https://doi.org/10.1080/15402002.2014.963583

18 Wright, S. T., Kerr, C. W., Doroszczuk, N. M., Kuszczak, S. M., Hang, P. C., & Luczkiewicz, D. L. (2014). The impact of dreams of the deceased on bereavement: a survey of hospice caregivers. *The American Journal of Hospice & Palliative Care, 31*(2), 132-138.

19 Black, J., Murkar, A., & Black, J. (2014, April 7). Examining the healing process through dreams in bereavement. *Sleep and Hypnosis, 16*(1-2), 10-17.

20 Kuiken, D., Dunn, S., & LoVerso, T. (2008). Expressive writing about dreams that follow trauma and loss. Dreaming, 18(2), 77–93.

21 Wray, T. J., & Price, A. B. (2005). *Grief dreams: How they help heal us after the death of a loved one.* San Francisco, CA: Jossey-Bass. P2

22 Wray, T. J., & Price, A. B. (2005). *Grief dreams: How they help heal us after the death of a loved one.* San Francisco, CA: Jossey-Bass.

23 Wray, T. J., & Price, A. B. (2005). *Grief dreams: How they help heal us after the death of a loved one.* San Francisco, CA: Jossey-Bass.

24 Zisook, S., & Shear, K. (2009, June). Grief and bereavement: what psychiatrists need to know. *World Psychiatry, 8*(2). Retrieved from https://www.ncbi.nlm.nih.gov/pmc/articles/PMC2691160/

25 Longfellow, H. W. (2000). *Longfellow poems and other writings.* J. D. McClatchy (Ed.). New York, NY: Penguin.

26 Wood, F. B. (2008, September). Helping young children cope. *Young Children, 63*(5), 28-31.

27 Bugge, K. E., Darbyshire, P., Rokholt, E. G., Haugstvedt, K. T., & Helseth, S. (2014). Young children's grief: Parents' understanding and coping . *Death Studies, 38*(1), 36-43. https://doi.org/10.1080/0 7481187.2012.718037

28 Ener, L., & Ray, D.C. (2018). Exploring characteristics of children presenting to counseling for grief and loss. *Journal of Child and Family Studies , 27*(), 860-871. https://doi.org/10.1007/s10826-017-0939-6

29 Krupnick, J. L. (1984). CHAPTER 5 Bereavement During Childhood and Adolescence. In *Bereavement Reactions, Consequences, and Care.* https://doi.org/10.17226/8

30 Pachur, T., Hertwig, R., & Steinmann, F. (2012). How do people judge risks: availability heuristic, affect heuristic, or both? *Journal of Experimental Psychology: Applied, 18*(3), 314-330. https://doi. org/10.1037/a0028279

31 Kakar, V., & Oberoi, N. (2016). Mourning with social media: Rewiring grief. *Indian Journal of Positive Psychology, 7*(3), 371-375.

32 Kakar, V., & Oberoi, N. (2016). Mourning with social media: Rewiring grief. *Indian Journal of Positive Psychology, 7*(3), 371-375.

33 Willis, E., & Ferrucci, P. (2017). Mourning and grief on Facebook: An examination of motivations for interacting with the deceased. *OMEGA- Journal of Death and Dying , 76*(2), 122-140. P124

34 Pennington, N. (2017). Tie strength and time: Mourning on social networking sites. *Journal of Broadcasting & Electronic Media, 61*(1), 11-23.

35 Hampton, K., & Wellman, B. (2003). Neighboring in netville: How the Internet supports community and social capital in a wired suburb. *City & Community*, *2*(4), 277-311.

36 Kakar, V., & Oberoi, N. (2016). Mourning with social media: Rewiring grief. *Indian Journal of Positive Psychology*, *7*(3), 371-375.

37 Pennington, N. (2017). Tie strength and time: Mourning on social networking sites. *Journal of Broadcasting & Electronic Media*, *61*(1), 11-23.

38 Falconer, K., Sachsenweger, M., Gibson, K., & Norman, H. (2011). Grieving in the internet age. *New Zealand Journal of Psychology*, *40*(3), 79-87.

39 Pennington, N. (2017). Tie strength and time: Mourning on social networking sites. *Journal of Broadcasting & Electronic Media*, *61*(1), 11-23.

40 Doug Flutie's parents die within an hour of each other. (2015). Retrieved from https://www.usatoday.com/story/sports/nfl/2015/11/18/doug-flutie-parents-die-dick-joan/76011882/

41 Takotsubo cardiomyopathy (broken-heart syndrome). (2018). Retrieved from https://www.health.harvard.edu/heart-health/takotsubo-cardiomyopathy-broken-heart-syndrome

42 Sifferlin, A. (2014). How grief makes you sick in old age. Retrieved from http://time.com/3311270/how-grief-makes-you-sick-in-old-age/

43 Elwert, F., & Christakis, N. (2008, November). The effect of widowhood on mortality by the causes of death of both spouses. *American Journal of Public Health, 98*(11). https://doi.org/10.2105/AJPH.2007.114348

44 Dahlstrom, L. (2008). Never to part: Devoted couples share life, death. Retrieved from http://www.nbcnews.com/id/26980587/ns/health-aging/t/never-part-devoted-couples-share-life-death/#.XLknPehKiUl

45 Schultze-Florey, C. R., Martinez-Maza, O., Magpantay, L., Breen, E. C., Irwin, M. R., Gundel, H., & O'Connor, M. (2012). When grief makes you sick: Bereavement induced systemic inflammation is a question of genotype. *Brain, Behavior, and Immunity, 26*(7), 1066-1071.

46 Lewis, C. S. (1961). *A Grief Observed.* New York, NY: HarperCollins.

47 Rosenfeld, E. (2018). The fire that changed the way we think about grief. Retrieved from https://www.thecrimson.com/article/2018/11/29/erich-lindemann-cocoanut-grove-fire-grief/

48 Lindemann, E. (1994, June). Symptomatology and management of acute grief. *American Journal of Psychiatry, 151*(6).

49 Lindemann, E. (1994, June). Symptomatology and management of acute grief. *American Journal of Psychiatry,* 151(6).

50 Vlemincx, E., Van Diest, I., & Van den Bergh, O. (2015). Emotion, sighing, and respiratory variability. *Psychophysiology, 52*(5), 657–666. https://doi.org/10.1111/psyp.12396

51 Tedeschi, R. G., & Calhoun, L. G. (2004). Posttraumatic Growth: Conceptual Foundations and Empirical Evidence. *Psychological Inquiry*, 15(1), 1–18.

52 Rosenfeld, E. (2018). The fire that changed the way we think about grief. Retrieved from https://www.thecrimson.com/article/2018/11/29/erich-lindemann-cocoanut-grove-fire-grief/

53 Rendon, J. (2015). How trauma can change you—For the better. Retrieved from http://time.com/3967885/how-trauma-can-change-you-for-the-better/

54 Tedeschi, R. G., & Calhoun, L. G. (2004). Posttraumatic Growth: Conceptual Foundations and Empirical Evidence. *Psychological Inquiry*, 15(1), 1–18.

55 Eschner, K. (2017). Three medical breakthroughs that can be traced back to a tragic nightclub fire. Retrieved from https://www.smithsonianmag.com/smart-news/three-medical-breakthroughs-can-be-traced-back-tragic-cocoanut-grove-fire-180967323/

56 Frankl, V. (2006). *Man's search for meaning*. Boston Massachusetts: Beacon Press.

57 Krause, N., Hayward, R. D., Bruce, R. D., & Woolever, C. (2014). Gratitude to God, Self-rated Health, and Depressive Symptoms. *Journal for the Scientific Study of Religion*, 53(2), 341-355.

58 Emmons, R. A., & McCullough, M. E. (2003). Counting blessings versus burdens: An experimental investigation of gratitude and subjective well-being in daily life. *Journal of personality and Social Psychology*, 84(2), 377-389. https://doi.org/10.1037/0022-3514.84.2.377

59 Ziglar, Z. (n.d.). The gratitude journey. Retrieved from https://www.ziglar.com/articles/the-gratitude-journey/ para 1

60 Zahn, R., Garrido, G., Moll, J., & Grafman, J. (2014). Individual differences in posterior cortical volume correlate with proneness to pride and gratitude. Social Cognitive and Affective Neuroscience, 9(11), 1676–1683.

61 Chowdhury, M. R. (2019). The Neuroscience of Gratitude and How It Affects Anxiety & Grief. Retrieved from https://positivepsychology.com/neuroscience-of-gratitude/

62 University of California - Los Angeles. (2009). Meditation increases brain gray matter. Retrieved from https://medicalxpress.com/news/2009-05-meditation-brain-gray.html

63 Bertocci, P. A., & Millard, R. M. (1963). *Personality and the good: Psychological and ethical perspectives*. New York: David McKay. p389

64 McCullough, M. E., Emmons, R. A., & Tsang, J. (2002). The grateful disposition: A conceptual and empirical topography. *Journal of Personality and Social Psychology, 82*(1), 112-127.

65 Donaldson, A. L. (1915, November 21). Trudeau's Life a Rare Romance in Medicine; A Hopeless Sufferer from Tuberculosis, He Found in the Adirondacks the Secret of Conquering the Disease and Became a Healer of Thousands. *New York Times*. Retrieved from https://localwiki.org/hsl/Edward_Livingston_Trudeau

66 Abraham Verghese receives national humanities medal. (n.d.). Retrieved from https://abrahamverghese.com/

67 Frankl, V. (2006). *Man's search for meaning*. Boston Massachusetts: Beacon Press.